T0259482

Sports Cardiology

Editor

MATTHEW W. MARTINEZ

CARDIOLOGY CLINICS

www.cardiology.theclinics.com

Editorial Board
JAMIL A. ABOULHOSN
DAVID M. SHAVELLE
TERRENCE D. WELCH
AUDREY H. WU

February 2023 • Volume 41 • Number 1

ELSEVIER

1600 John F. Kennedy Boulevard • Suite 1800 • Philadelphia, Pennsylvania, 19103-2899

http://www.theclinics.com

CARDIOLOGY CLINICS Volume 41, Number 1
February 2023 ISSN 0733-8651, ISBN-13: 978-0-323-96189-9

Editor: Joanna Collett
Developmental Editor: Karen Justine Solomon

© **2023 Elsevier Inc. All rights reserved.**

This periodical and the individual contributions contained in it are protected under copyright by Elsevier, and the following terms and conditions apply to their use:

Photocopying
Single photocopies of single articles may be made for personal use as allowed by national copyright laws. Permission of the Publisher and payment of a fee is required for all other photocopying, including multiple or systematic copying, copying for advertising or promotional purposes, resale, and all forms of document delivery. Special rates are available for educational institutions that wish to make photocopies for non-profit educational classroom use. For information on how to seek permission visit www.elsevier.com/permissions or call: (+44) 1865 843830 (UK)/(+1) 215 239 3804 (USA).

Derivative Works
Subscribers may reproduce tables of contents or prepare lists of articles including abstracts for internal circulation within their institutions. Permission of the Publisher is required for resale or distribution outside the institution. Permission of the Publisher is required for all other derivative works, including compilations and translations (please consult www.elsevier.com/permissions).

Electronic Storage or Usage
Permission of the Publisher is required to store or use electronically any material contained in this periodical, including any article or part of an article (please consult www.elsevier.com/permissions). Except as outlined above, no part of this publication may be reproduced, stored in a retrieval system or transmitted in any form or by any means, electronic, mechanical, photo-copying, recording or otherwise, without prior written permission of the Publisher.

Notice
No responsibility is assumed by the Publisher for any injury and/or damage to persons or property as a matter of products liability, negligence or otherwise, or from any use or operation of any methods, products, instructions or ideas contained in the material herein. Because of rapid advances in the medical sciences, in particular, independent verification of diagnoses and drug dosages should be made.

Although all advertising material is expected to conform to ethical (medical) standards, inclusion in this publication does not constitute a guarantee or endorsement of the quality or value of such product or of the claims made of it by its manufacturer.

Cardiology Clinics (ISSN 0733-8651) is published quarterly by Elsevier Inc., 360 Park Avenue South, New York, NY 10010-1710. Months of issue are February, May, August, and November. Business and Editorial Offices: 1600 John F. Kennedy Blvd., Ste. 1800, Philadelphia, PA 19103-2899. Customer Service Office: 3251 Riverport Lane, Maryland Heights, MO 63043. Periodicals post-age paid at New York, NY and additional mailing offices. Subscription prices are $377.00 per year for US individuals, $743.00 per year for US institutions, $100.00 per year for US students and residents, $468.00 per year for Canadian individuals, $932.00 per year for Canadian institutions, $490.00 per year for international individuals, $932.00 per year for international institutions, $100.00 per year for Canadian students/residents and $220.00 per year for international students/residents. To receive student/resident rate, orders must be accompanied by name of affiliated institution, data of term, and the *signature* of program/residency coordinator on institution letterhead. Orders will be billed at individual rate until proof of status is received. Foreign air speed delivery is included in all *Clinics* subscription prices. All prices are subject to change without notice. **POSTMASTER:** Send address changes to *Cardiology Clinics*, Elsevier Health Sciences Division, Subscription Customer Service, 3251 Riverport Lane, Maryland Heights, MO 63043. **Customer Service: 1-800-654-2452 (U.S. and Canada); 314-447-8871 (outside U.S. and Canada). Fax: 314-447-8029. E-mail: journalscus-tomerservice-usa@elsevier.com (for print support); journalsonlinesupport-usa@elsevier.com (for online support).**

Reprints. For copies of 100 or more, of articles in this publication, please contact the Commercial Reprints Department, Elsevier Inc., 360 Park Avenue South, New York, NY 10010-1710. Tel.: 212-633-3874; Fax: 212-633-3820; E-mail: reprints@elsevier.com.

Cardiology Clinics is also published in Spanish by McGraw-Hill Interamericana Editores S. A., P.O. Box 5-237, 06500, Mexico D. F., Mexico; in Portuguese by Reichmann and Alfonso Editores Rio de Janeiro, Brazil; and in Greek by Dimitrios P. Lagos, 8 Pondon Street, GR115-28 Ilissia, Greece.

Cardiology Clinics is covered in *MEDLINE/PubMed (Index Medicus), Excerpta Medica, The Cumulative Index to Nursing and Allied Health Literature* (CINAHL).

Contributors

EDITORIAL BOARD

JAMIL A. ABOULHOSN, MD, FACC, FSCAI
Director, Ahmanson/UCLA Adult Congenital
Heart Center, Streisand/American Heart
Association Endowed Chair, Divisions of
Cardiology and Pediatric Cardiology, David
Geffen School of Medicine at UCLA, Los
Angeles, California, USA

DAVID M. SHAVELLE, MD, FACC, FSCAI
Associate Professor, Keck School of Medicine
of USC, Director, General Cardiovascular
Fellowship Program, Director, Cardiac
Catheterization Laboratory, LAC + USC
Medical Center, Division of Cardiovascular
Medicine, University of Southern California,
Los Angeles, California, USA; MemorialCare
Heart and Vascular Institute, Long Beach
Medical Center, Long Beach, California, USA

TERRENCE D. WELCH, MD, FACC
Associate Professor of Medicine and Medical
Education, Director, Cardiovascular Fellowship
Program, Section of Cardiovascular Medicine,
Dartmouth-Hitchcock Heart and Vascular
Center, Lebanon, New Hampshire, USA;
Dartmouth Geisel School of Medicine,
Hanover, New Hampshire, USA

AUDREY H. WU, MD, MPH
Associate Professor, Advanced Heart Failure
and Transplant Program, Division of
Cardiovascular Medicine, Department of
Medicine, University of Michigan, Ann Arbor,
Michigan, USA

EDITOR

MATTHEW W. MARTINEZ, MD
Director of Sports Cardiology and
Hypertrophic Cardiomyopathy Program, Co-
Director, Chanin T. Mast Hypertrophic

Cardiomyopathy Center and Sports
Cardiology, Atlantic Health System/Morristown
Medical Center, Department of Cardiology,
Morristown, New Jersey, USA

AUTHORS

ROBYN E. BRYDE, MD
Department of Cardiovascular Medicine, Mayo
Clinic, Jacksonville, Florida, USA

TIMOTHY W. CHURCHILL, MD
Division of Cardiology, Massachusetts General
Hospital, Cardiovascular Performance
Program, Massachusetts General Hospital

LESLIE T. COOPER Jr, MD
Department of Cardiovascular Medicine, Mayo
Clinic, Jacksonville, Florida, USA

PETER N. DEAN, MD
Division of Pediatric Cardiology, Department of
Pediatrics, University of Virginia,
Charlottesville, Virginia, USA

DAMIAN N. DI FLORIO, BS
PhD Student, Department of Cardiovascular
Medicine, Mayo Clinic, Jacksonville, Florida,
USA; Center for Clinical and Translational
Science, Mayo Clinic, Rochester, Minnesota,
USA

ELIZABETH H. DINEEN, DO
Assistant Professor of Medicine and
Cardiology, University of California Irvine
Medical Center, Orange, California, USA

TAM DOAN, MD
Assistant Professor of Pediatrics, Division of
Pediatric Cardiology, Coronary Artery
Anomalies Program, The Lillie Frank
Abercrombie Section of Cardiology, Texas
Children's Hospital, Baylor College of
Medicine, Houston, Texas, USA

JONATHAN A. DREZNER, MD
University of Washington Medical Center for
Sports Cardiology, Massachusetts General
Hospital

JAMIE EDWARDS, MSc
School of Psychology and Life Sciences,
Canterbury Christ Church University, Kent,
United Kingdom

MICHAEL S. EMERY, MD, MS
Sports Cardiology Center, Department of
Cardiovascular Medicine, Heart, Vascular

DELISA FAIRWEATHER, PhD
Department of Cardiovascular Medicine, Mayo
Clinic, Jacksonville, Florida, USA; Center for
Clinical and Translational Science, Mayo Clinic,
Rochester, Minnesota, USA

MARK C. HAIGNEY, MD
Director, Military Cardiovascular Outcomes
Research, Professor of Medicine and
Pharmacology, Uniformed Services University,
Bethesda, Maryland, USA

MUSTAFA HUSAINI, MD
Department of Medicine, Division of
Cardiovascular Medicine, Washington
University School of Medicine, St Louis,
Missouri, USA

LANIER B. JACKSON, MD
Division of Pediatric Cardiology, Department of
Pediatrics, Medical University of South
Carolina, Charleston, South Carolina, USA

BRADLEY KAY, MD
Section of Cardiovascular Medicine, Yale
School of Medicine, New Haven, Connecticut,
USA

JONATHAN H. KIM, MD, MSc
Division of Cardiology, Emory Clinical
Cardiovascular Research Institute, Emory
University School of Medicine, Atlanta,
Georgia, USA

RACHEL LAMPERT, MD
Professor of Medicine, Section of
Cardiovascular Medicine, Yale School of
Medicine, New Haven, Connecticut, USA

BENJAMIN D. LEVINE, MD
Director, Institute for Exercise and
Environmental Medicine, Professor of
Medicine and Cardiology, The University of
Texas Southwestern Medical Center, Dallas,
Texas, USA

MATTHEW W. MARTINEZ, MD
Director of Sports Cardiology and
Hypertrophic Cardiomyopathy Program, Co-
Director, Chanin T. Mast Hypertrophic
Cardiomyopathy Center and Sports
Cardiology, Atlantic Health System/Morristown
Medical Center, Department of Cardiology,
Morristown, New Jersey, USA

SILVANA MOLOSSI, MD, PhD
Associate Professor of Pediatrics, Division of
Pediatric Cardiology, Coronary Artery
Anomalies Program, The Lillie Frank
Abercrombie Section of Cardiology, Texas
Children's Hospital, Baylor College of
Medicine, Houston, Texas, USA

JAMIE O'DRISCOLL, PhD
School of Psychology and Life Sciences,
Canterbury Christ Church University, Kent,
United Kingdom

MICHAEL PAPADAKIS, MD
Cardiovascular Clinical Academic Group, St
George's, University of London, London,
United Kingdom

BRADLEY J. PETEK, MD
Division of Cardiology, Cardiovascular
Performance Program, Massachusetts
General Hospital

TRISTAN RAMCHARAN, MD
Heart Unit, Birmingham Children's Hospital,
Birmingham, United Kingdom; MSc Sports
Cardiology, St George's, University of London,
London, United Kingdom

ANDREW M. REITTINGER, MD
Division of Pediatric Cardiology, Department of
Pediatrics, University of Virginia,
Charlottesville, Virginia, USA

SHAGUN SACHDEVA, MD
Assistant Professor of Pediatrics, Division of
Pediatric Cardiology, Coronary Artery
Anomalies Program, The Lillie Frank
Abercrombie Section of Cardiology, Texas

Children's Hospital, Baylor College of
Medicine, Houston, Texas, USA

JASON V. TSO, MD
Division of Cardiology, Emory University
School of Medicine, Atlanta, Georgia, USA

JENNIFER XU, MD
Cardiology Fellow, University of California
Irvine Medical Center, Orange, California, USA

Contents

for ECG interpretation in athletes, the International Criteria, was developed to distinguish physiologic from pathologic ECG findings in athletes. Although application of the International Criteria has reduced the PPCS false-positive rate, interpretative challenges and potential areas of improvement remain. This review provides an overview of common pitfalls and future directions for ECG interpretation in athletes.

Congenital coronary anomalies are not an infrequent occurrence and their clinical presentation typically occurs during early years, though may be manifested only in adulthood. In the setting of anomalous aortic origin of a coronary artery, this is particularly concerning as it inflicts sudden loss of healthy young lives. Risk stratification remains a challenge and so does the best management decision-making in these patients, particularly if asymptomatic. Standardized approach to evaluation and management, with careful data collection and collaboration among centers, will likely impact future outcomes in this patient population, thus allowing for exercise participation and healthier lives.

The noninvasive assessment of oxygen consumption, carbon dioxide production, and ventilation during a cardiopulmonary exercise test (CPET) provides insight into the cardiovascular, pulmonary, and metabolic system's ability to respond to exercise. Exercise physiology has been shown to be distinct for competitive athletes and highly active persons (CAHAPs), thus creating more nuanced interpretations of CPET parameters. CPET in CAHAP is an important test that can be used for both diagnosis (provoking symptoms during a truly maximal test) and performance.

Until recently, implantable cardioverter defibrillators (ICDs) were considered a contraindication to competitive athletics. Recent prospective observational registry data in athletes with ICDs who participated in sports against the societal recommendations at the time have demonstrated the safety of sports participation. While athletes did receive both appropriate and inappropriate shocks, these were not more frequent during sports participation than other activity, and there were no sports-related deaths or need for external resuscitation in the 440 athlete cohort (median followup 44 months). Optimization of medical therapies, device settings and having an emergency action plan allow many athletes to safely continue athletic activity.

Tactical athletes are individuals in the military, law enforcement, and other professions whose occupations have significant physical fitness requirements coupled with the potential for exposure to life-threatening situations. Such exposures can have varied hemodynamic effects on the cardiovascular system. It is crucial that their clinical evaluation is inclusive of specific occupational requirements. Safety protocols regarding medical clearance are relatively more stringent for this population than for competitive athletes due to the increased impact to the tactical athlete, their team, and the population they aim to serve and protect should they experience a cardiovascular event on the job.

Myocarditis is an inflammatory disease of the myocardium secondary to infectious and noninfectious insults. The most feared consequence of myocarditis is sudden cardiac death owing to electrical instability and arrhythmia. Typical presenting symptoms include chest pain, dyspnea, palpitations and/or heart failure. Diagnosis is usually made with history, electrocardiogram, biomarkers, echocardiogram, and cardiac MRI (CMR). Application of the Lake Louise criteria to CMR results can help identify cases of myocarditis. Treatment is usually supportive with medical therapy, and patients are recommended to abstain from exercise for 3 to 6 months. Exercise restrictions may be lifted after normalization on follow-up testing.

CARDIOLOGY CLINICS

SERIES OF RELATED INTEREST

Cardiac Electrophysiology Clinics
Available at: https://www.cardiacep.theclinics.com/
Heart Failure Clinics
Available at: https://www.heartfailure.theclinics.com/
Interventional Cardiology Clinics
Available at: https://www.interventional.theclinics.com/

Preface

Sports Cardiology: Athlete Risk Identification, Assessment, and Risk Mitigation

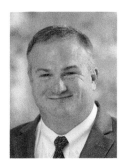

Matthew W. Martinez, MD
Editor

Cardiovascular causes account for most sports-related deaths, especially in young athletes. Causes of sudden cardiac arrest are heterogeneous and associated with a spectrum of cardiovascular diseases. Most cases are associated with congenital or acquired cardiac abnormalities, with most events in individuals that had not been previously detected. The field of sports and exercise cardiology continues to evolve to encompass the burgeoning number of people who are physically active, including tactical athletes, and those with cardiovascular diseases or risk factors. Sports Cardiologists are tasked to work with other sports medicine providers to identify those at risk, manage those with known cardiovascular risk factors, and develop methods for prevention of sudden cardiac arrest. Development of preparticipation evaluations for all prospective athletes and for individuals at risk for or with known cardiac disease has been employed to mitigate risk. Currently, there are numerous national and international guidelines and clinical tools available to help physicians provide cardiovascular care for their athletic patients. These resources address preparticipation screening (primary prevention) recommendations and tools to identify athletes at possible increased risk of sudden cardiac arrest; secondary evaluation for suspected cardiovascular conditions; and management, participation eligibility criteria, and return to play for individuals with known cardiovascular conditions. Some of those recommendations are in need of an update. As we see continued focus on the role of the Sports Cardiologist as a valued member of the athlete's medical team, we see research following this growth. The accompanying articles update readers on state-of-the-art issues that are germane to the practicing Sports Cardiologist.

Matthew W. Martinez, MD
Atlantic Health System/
Morristown Medical Center
Department of Cardiology
111 Madison Avenue
Suite 301
Morristown, NJ 07960, USA

E-mail address:
matthew.martinez@atlantichealth.org

https://doi.org/10.1016/j.ccl.2022.10.001
0733-8651/23/© 2022 Published by Elsevier Inc.

cardiology.theclinics.com

Preface

Sports Cardiology: Athlete
Risk Stratification,
Assessment, and Risk
Mitigation

Preparticipation Cardiac Evaluation from the Pediatric Perspective

Andrew M. Reittinger, MD[a], Lanier B. Jackson, MD[b], Peter N. Dean, MD[a],*

KEYWORDS

- Preparticipation examination • Sudden cardiac death • Sports cardiology • Pediatric • Adolescent

KEY POINTS

- The sports preparticipation examination is an opportunity to screen for risk factors for sudden cardiac death (SCD).
- Evaluation of the pediatric population presents different considerations and challenges compared with adults.
- A normal preparticipation or cardiac examination does not mean that it will be normal in perpetuity, as the age of onset of certain cardiac disorders predisposing to SCD present at varying times during development.

INTRODUCTION

Each year millions of children and adolescents undergo sports preparticipation evaluations (PPEs) before participating in organized sports. The clinicians who evaluate these patients have a wide range of expertise and experience performing sports PPEs and/or evaluating pediatric and adolescent patients. This article is designed to summarize the current thoughts on the PPE with a specific slant toward the pediatric and early adolescent evaluations and how they may differ from those in adults.

CASES

1. An 11-year-old boy presents for sports clearance to play high school basketball. He has a family medical history of hypertrophic cardiomyopathy (HCM) in his father. His father has not had genetic testing. **Figs. 1** and **2** show his normal electrocardiogram (ECG) and normal echocardiogram. What do you do next?

2. A 10-year-old boy presents for clearance before youth league soccer. When asked about a history of syncope or unresponsive spells, his mother reports he had a recent syncopal episode. She reports that he was running to the school bus with his siblings when she noticed that he started to lag behind his siblings, fell to his knees, screamed, and then fell on his face. He was noted to be unconscious for a period of about 15 seconds and did not require any resuscitative measures. He was noted to have significant abrasions on his face. When he recovered, he apologized for the fact that "his legs stopped working." His mother recounts that 2 months earlier she received a call from school after he fell while running on the track during gym class. This event was also associated facial abrasions. His mother attributed the inability to catch himself during his fall to prevent facial injury to what she described as general clumsiness and his history of mild gross motor delay. What do you do next?

3. An 18-year-old male college baseball player presents to a mass preparticipation screening clinic. He reports a history of Kawasaki disease (KD) and is currently taking aspirin and dipyridamole. There is no access to outside medical records. What do you do next?

a Division of Pediatric Cardiology, Department of Pediatrics, University of Virginia, 1204 West Main Street, Battle Building, 6th Floor, Charlottesville, VA 22903, USA; b Division of Pediatric Cardiology, Department of Pediatrics, Medical University of South Carolina, 10 McClennan Banks Drive, MSC 915, Charleston, SC 29425, USA
* Corresponding author.
E-mail address: PND8J@hscmail.mcc.virginia.edu

Cardiol Clin 41 (2023) 1–14
https://doi.org/10.1016/j.ccl.2022.08.001
0733-8651/23/© 2022 Elsevier Inc. All rights reserved.

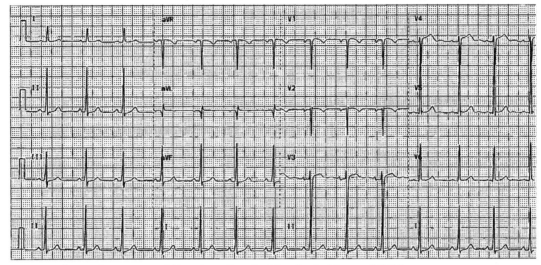

Fig. 1. Initial ECG of an 11-year-old boy from Case 1 with a family history of HCM.

WHAT IS THE PURPOSE OF PREPARTICIPATION EVALUATION?

The purpose of preparticipation screening is to identify individuals who may be at risk for adverse health effects such as illness or injury secondary to sports participation. The most serious potential adverse event is sudden cardiac arrest (SCA) or sudden cardiac death (SCD). As SCA and SCD can sometimes be the first presentation of an underlying cardiac condition, the PPE is an attempt to catch underlying cardiac diseases that predispose individuals to SCA and SCD.

Although studies have called into question the efficacy of the PPE and in particular the screening tools for SCA risk factors,[1] the PPE is still viewed as an avenue to encourage non-acute primary care visits.[2] This gives the opportunity to provide counseling on not only sports-related physical

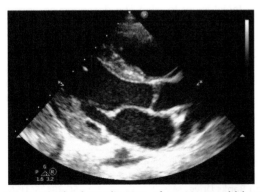

Fig. 2. Initial echocardiogram of an 11-year-old boy from Case 1 with a family history of HCM. This is a parasternal long axis image in 2D showing normal left ventricular and interventricular septal dimensions.

concerns but also mental health topics, diet, high-risk behaviors, and medication, supplement illicit drug use.

Although overall the evaluation is similar to the adult population, there are some differences and particular challenges in the pediatric population. The authors intend to focus on these in this article.

DIFFERENCES IN INCIDENCE AND CAUSES OF SUDDEN CARDIAC ARREST

In order to perform an appropriate PPE the clinician should know the conditions that predispose athletes to SCA or SCD. The conditions that cause SCA are one of the differences in children and adolescents compared with adults.

Overall, the incidence of SCA in adults is approximately 135 per 100,000,[3] with coronary artery disease accounting for 75% to 80% of SCD in the United States and Europe. Fortunately, in the young adult population, the rate of SCD is significantly lower (0.7 per 100,000 person-years in 18–35 year old group and 13.7 per 100,000 person-years in those over 35 years of age).[4]

Specifically looking at athletes, the incidence of sports-related sudden death in young athletes is 0.5 to 2.1 per 100,000 people per year.[4] This is higher in elite athletes. The incidence of SCD over a 4-year collegiate athletic career in the United States in any sport is 1:13,425 based on data gathered from the National Collegiate Athletic Association (NCAA). The risk seems to be higher in males and black athletes. Basketball (male and female) was the sport with the highest rate of SCD, followed by men's soccer and men's football. Division I male basketball players had the highest incidence of SCD at 1:5200 athlete years. The common causes of SCD in the NCAA population were autopsy-negative sudden unexplained death (25%), verified or suspected cardiomyopathy (24%; 8% confirmed HCM), coronary artery anomalies or disease (21%), and myocarditis (10%). In total, SCD comprised 15% of sudden death in NCAA athletes, whereas the combination of accidents, homicide, and suicide accounted for 68%.[5]

A recent study by Burns and colleagues looked into the incidence and cause of sudden death in the pediatric population. The 2020 study found the incidence of sudden death was 1.9 per 100,000 in children between 1 and 17 years of age. The lowest incidence was in 6 to 9 year olds (1.1/100,000 children), and the highest incidence was in 14 to 17 year olds (2.4/100,000). Unfortunately, it was difficult to determine the cause of sudden death in a significant number of cases (43% of the cases were "unexplained"). Cardiac causes accounted for 16% of the "explained" cases and were the second most common cause (behind respiratory). Only a small percentage of all sudden death events occurred cases occurred during exertional activities (13%).[6] These findings highlight that medical providers should be thinking of the variety of causes of sudden in all pediatric patients and not just "athletes."

Another epidemiologic study out of Denmark published in 2014 reports that the incidence of confirmed or suspected SCD in children 1 to 18 year old is 1.1 per 100,000 person-years (0.8 per 100,000 when suspected cases are excluded). In children older than 1 year, the incidence of SCD death increased to its highest levels in the 13 to 18 year old age group.[7] Of the SCDs, only 23% had previously diagnosed cardiac disorders, and 61% were not known to have any health conditions. After autopsy, 70% of deaths were thought to be cardiac in origin with myocarditis being the highest incidence at 9%. In this population, only 59% of patients experienced symptoms before the SCD.[7]

DIFFERENCES IN PHENOTYPE PRESENTATION

Another significant difference between adults and pediatric patients is pediatric patients are more likely to be evaluated before their phenotype has presented. Although some cardiac conditions that predispose to SCA will be present at birth (Wolff–Parkinson–White, long QT syndrome [LQTS], anomalous origin of a coronary artery, aortic valve stenosis, and so forth), there are others that cannot be diagnosed early in life

even with appropriate or extensive cardiac testing.

HCM is a leading cause of sudden death in young athletes,[8] but screening for HCM can be difficult at young ages because sometimes the phenotype is not present until adulthood.[9] Patients at risk for developing HCM may have normal testing early in childhood and then develop HCM and be at risk for SCD later in adolescents. Owing to this, it is recommended that children who are asymptomatic who have a first-degree relative with HCM should be screened with an ECG and echocardiogram every 1 to 3 years.[9]

Marfan syndrome is similar to HCM in that individuals can have relatively normal physical examinations and normal sized aortic roots in childhood but develop significant aortic dilation throughout adolescence and young adulthood, predisposing them to aortic root dissection and rupture. Recent studies looking at the phenotypes of patients with pathologic genetic mutations for Marfan syndrome showed that only 56% of 10 to 18 year olds will meet the clinical diagnostic criteria for Marfan[10] compared with 79% of adults.[11]

Arrhythmogenic right ventricular cardiomyopathy (ARVC) is another cause of SCA that has variable ages of presentation. ARVC is particularly challenging to diagnosis in the pediatric population as there is typically a "concealed phase," during which no structural or electrocardiographic abnormalities are identifiable but malignant arrhythmias with sports or physical activity can occur.[12] Studies have demonstrated that pediatric patients are more likely than adults to have SCA as their presenting symptom for this reason.[13,14] Unfortunately, diagnosis can be challenging.[15] In a recent study, even pediatric patients who were thought to have definitive ARVC after a cardiac MRI rarely had abnormal ECGs (4%) and none had abnormal echocardiograms.[16]

Because of the variable presentations of many cardiac diseases over time, providers evaluating patients in early or mid-childhood need to understand the limits of their screening and consider repeat testing later in adolescence or young adulthood, regardless of whether the initial screening included cardiac testing. Similarly, providers should be cognizant of the fact that in some circumstances, the parents or other first-degree relatives of a young athlete are themselves of an age at which potential cardiac disorders have not clinically presented.

Providers need to stress to patients and families that a "normal cardiac screen" demonstrates that there is no evidence of cardiac disease at that specific point in time. This designation does not last in

Table 1
Possible differences between pediatric and young adult/adult preparticipation cardiac screening

Pediatric Specific Screening	Young Adult and Adult Screening
More likely to have vague or unclear symptoms	Better able to communicate symptoms
Likely requires repeat screening as adolescent and/or young adult	More likely to have already expressed the phenotype of specific cardiac disease
Parents too young to demonstrate phenotype	Older parents with more detail about family history
Pediatric providers are less experienced in ECGs	Family physicians and adult providers more experienced interpreting ECGs
More likely to have undiagnosed congenital heart disease	Less likely to have undiagnosed congenital heart disease
More likely to have history of Kawasaki disease	
Suboptimal criteria for ECG abnormalities	

perpetuity and new cardiac symptoms or concerns should be reevaluated. Patients under the assumption that their heart is "normal" may not seek medical care for otherwise concerning cardiac symptoms.

This is highlighted by a recent article that showed that the rate of SCD in 11,168 adolescent soccer players was still 6.8 per 100,000 despite extensive cardiac screening (history, examination, ECG, and echocardiogram) before participation. The reason for the relatively high number of SCD was related to cardiomyopathies that were not detected by screening. The mean age of screening was 16.4 ± 1.2 years, and the time between the screening and the episode of SCD was 6.8 years.[17] Although it is certainly unknown whether athletes would have had detectable abnormalities around the time of the SCD, this suggests that serial screening may be indicated. In a response to a Letter to the Editor, the investigators of the study state that the English Football Association has recently recommended initial screening at 16 years of age as part of a fitness assessment before signing a professional contract and repeat screening 18, 20, and 25 year old (**Table 1**) greater than.[17]

WHO SHOULD BE EVALUATED AND WHEN SHOULD IT START?

As most adults are not still participating in competitive sports as they age, it seems easier to describe an adult as a competitive athlete, a recreational athlete, or a nonathlete. This is more difficult in the pediatric population, as sport intensity varies greatly and participation varies from year to year. Owing to this, it seems as though categorizing elementary school students or junior high students as an "athlete" or "nonathlete" is not a medically important classification. This is in line with the recent American Academy of Pediatrics (AAP)

policy statement on the topic of screening for sudden death.[18] In that statement, they recommend screening patients every 2 to 3 years without any differentiation between athlete and nonathlete. It also suggests that screening should be performed starting at age six. They recommend four specific questions:

1. Have you ever fainted, passed out, or had an unexplained seizure suddenly and without warning, especially during exercise or in response to sudden loud noises, such as doorbells, alarm clocks, and ringing telephones?
2. Have you ever had exercise-related chest pain or shortness of breath?
3. Has anyone in your immediate family (parents, grandparents, siblings) or other, more distant relatives (aunts, uncles, cousins) died of heart problems or had an unexpected sudden death before age 50? This would include unexpected drownings, unexplained auto crashes in which the relative was driving, or sudden infant death syndrome (SIDS).
4. Are you related to anyone with HCM or hypertrophic obstructive cardiomyopathy, Marfan syndrome, arrhythmogenic cardiomyopathy, LQTS, short QT syndrome, Brugada Syndrome, or catecholaminergic polymorphic ventricular tachycardia or anyone younger than 50 years with a pacemaker or implantable defibrillator?[15]

The first two questions are likely not useful for children under 6 year old, but the last two questions, regarding family history are important at any age. LQTS and HCM are causes of SIDS or death in early childhood, so obtaining a detailed family history is important even in infancy. The authors believe that primary care physicians should be asking those questions or similar questions starting at the well-child visits soon after birth.

As adolescents enter high school and college, the line between athletes and nonathletes becomes better demarcated, but it still is not completely clear. Most of the sports participation is likely sanctioned through the school, but some elite-level or "travel" sports participants do not play on their corresponding school-sanctioned teams. Beyond this, there are certainly other physically demanding sports and activities undertaken by the teenager or young adult that are similar in their potential to cause SCA (hiking, climbing, mountain biking, skiing, trampolining, and so forth). Owing to this, primary care physicians should be asking questions about physical activity, cardiac symptoms with exertion, and family history regardless of whether or not there is an official "school preparticipation form" to sign. In a similar fashion, ECG screening programs, if offered, should be offered to any adolescent, regardless of their "athlete" status.

WHERE DO PREPARTICIPATION EVALUATIONS OCCUR?

Current PPE guidelines recommend yearly screening at least 6 weeks before the first sports practice or workout.[18] Ideally, these visits would occur with the patient's primary care provider, but there are other settings where evaluations occur, including mass screening events or urgent care offices. Most states require that a medical doctor, doctor of osteopathic medicine, nurse practitioner, or physician's assistant provide the clearance, but there is typically no discussion on experience or specific specialty of the provider.

The preferred provider is the patient's primary care provider. This allows for centralization of a patient's care, access to patient's past medical records, more nuanced understanding of the patient's medical, family, and social histories, and the ability to have consistent longitudinal follow-up. It also provides appropriate follow-up of referrals to ensure they are performed and recommendations are followed.

Although they are time efficient and allow for improved access to medical providers, mass screening events such as those in a school gymnasium can be problematic. These potential problems are (1) difficulty maintaining patient privacy and a safe space for patient to bring concerns to physician, (2) suboptimal environment for physical examination, (3) lack of access to patient's medical records, (4) lack of time and space for appropriate counseling when an abnormality or suspected abnormality is found, and (5) difficulty ensuring appropriate follow-up/referrals when abnormalities are found. The concept of mass PPE

events promotes efficiency, but could also unintentionally create the feeling of being rushed, which may alter a provider's typical practice or athlete's willingness to disclose symptoms. The potential problems with mass screenings are not a reason to avoid doing them, but they should be addressed.[18]

THE COMPONENTS OF THE PREPARTICIPATION EVALUATION

Typically, PPEs are based on the PPE monograph that has been developed and endorsed by the AAP, American Academy of Family Physicians, the American College of Sports Medicine, and American Medical Society for Sports Medicine for the past 40 years (AMSSM).[118] There is also an American Heart Association (AHA) 14-point questionnaire that has a similar format and questions.[19]

The PPE has three, and possibly four, main parts: history, family history, and examination and sometimes an ECG.

History

A medical history, encompassing both past medical history and cardiac symptoms, is an essential part of any patient encounter and should be carried out in any PPE. Cardiac symptoms with exercise should prompt further investigation. In addition, other odd or suspicious symptoms such as seizures, syncope, or extensive breath holding spells should be considered as potential signs of malignant arrhythmias. Any known or previously diagnosed cardiac pathology, including congenital heart disease, cardiac arrhythmia or channelopathies, cardiomyopathy, history of myocarditis, or coronary artery anomalies, including those caused by KD, should be evaluated by a cardiologist before clearance.

Studies have shown that complete agreement between athlete and parental reports of medical history on the PPE is less than 20%. The cardiovascular section, along with neurologic, musculoskeletal, and weight sections, accounted for nearly 60% of the discrepancies.[20] This highlights the importance of involving parents or primary caregivers in the history.

How to Respond When a History of Cardiac Disease Is Reported

Typically, when a patient reports a history of cardiac disease, they should be cleared by the cardiologist caring for that patient.

Providers evaluating pediatric athletes are more likely to be confronted with known congenital heart

Table 2 Common causes of cardiac and noncardiac pediatric chest pain	
Causes	Features
Cardiac chest pain	
Myocarditis	Nonspecific symptoms ranging from mild to signs of shock, often mimicking sepsis. Tachycardia and hypotension on vitals. ECG with diffuse ST-segment and T-wave abnormalities and often low voltages, particularly in precordial leads
Pericarditis	Retrosternal chest pain alleviated by leaning forward, often associated with fever or viral illness, friction rub on auscultation, ST-segment elevation, and PR depression on ECG
Aortic stenosis (AS)/coarctation (CoA)	Fatigue, dyspnea, angina, and syncope can be presenting symptoms, but only in more moderate to severe disease, blood pressure differentials (R arm > L arm in AS, R arm > either leg in CoA). Systolic murmur may be heard. Decreased lower extremity pulses in CoA
Ischemia	Anginal chest pain due to increased myocardial demand or decreased ability to supply the myocardium with its metabolic needs includes atherosclerotic coronary anomalies and

(continued on next page)

Table 2 (continued)	
Causes	Features
	acquired coronary artery disease from inflammatory causes such as Kawasaki disease and multisystem inflammatory syndrome in children
Mitral valve prolapse	May present with chest pain, anxiety, palpitations, or shortness of breath. Found in patients with connective tissue disorder. Associated with a mid-to-late systolic click with a high-pitched late systolic murmur
Arrhythmia	Supraventricular tachycardia or ventricular ectopy/tachycardia can cause chest pain, palpitations, diaphoresis, anxiety, shortness of breath, exercise intolerance, or pre-syncopal or syncopal symptoms. Will be tachycardic
Noncardiac chest pain	
Costochondritis	Reproducible pain on palpation and the costochondral junction
Precordial Catch	Sharp, localized pain that is brief and can be exacerbated with inspiration. Can often occur at test
Musculoskeletal	Associated with trauma or overuse. Can be seen frequently in athletes or those with recent respiratory

(continued on next page)

Table 2 (continued)	
Causes	Features
	infection featuring frequent cough
Asthma	Chest tightness and can be exercise-induced. Have trouble with inhalation and can have associated respiratory or allergic symptoms
Gastroesophageal reflux/ esophagitis	Epigastric pain with burning sensation. Can have associated regurgitation or metallic taste in the mouth. Symptoms worsened by certain types of food or exertion shortly after eating

disease or undiagnosed congenital heart disease. Often these congenital heart defects, repaired or unrepaired, do not have significant impact on sports participation. Examples of these include small atrial septal defects, small patent ductus arteriosus, mild pulmonary valve stenosis, repaired ventricular septal defects, among others. Sometimes the congenital heart disease is significant and can have significant implications for sports participation. Given this, when an athlete has congenital heart disease, they should be evaluated by a pediatric or congenital cardiologist before participation.

KD is an inflammatory disease of early childhood that can cause coronary artery aneurysms and subsequent coronary artery thrombus and stenosis. The huge majority of patients recover without significant coronary sequelae but some will have residual disease that may impact exercise and sports participation. As KD was only fully described in the mid to late 1970s and most patients recover without residual heart disease, providers who do not routinely care for pediatric patients may have limited experience. No exercise restrictions are indicated if patients did not have coronary artery abnormalities during the acute phase of KD or if they have had complete resolution of coronary aneurysms. If the athlete has persistent coronary artery aneurysms, antiplatelet or anticoagulation treatment is likely indicated

and they are at risk for developing coronary artery stenosis, both of which can impact decisions regarding sports participation.[21]

How to Respond to a History of Cardiac Symptoms

A report of cardiac symptoms by a patient is important because it can be a signal for the provider that cardiac disease is present. Reporting of symptoms can be challenging for any patient, but it can be especially difficult for children and adolescents. Owing to a lack of experience, a lack of vocabulary, and an intimidating environment, young patients are more likely to report vague symptoms or not fully understand or remember the situation when they had symptoms. Owing to these difficulties, providers asking and evaluating these symptoms should be experienced in interviewing pediatric and adolescent patients.

Chest pain

Chest pain is an extremely common complaint in the pediatric population—fortunately, only 0.2% to 1% of reported chest pain is cardiac in nature in the pediatric and adolescent population.[22] Red flags for cardiac chest pain include exertional pain and pain associated with palpitations or syncope (**Table 2**).

Syncope

Pre-syncope and syncope are frequently encountered in pediatric and adolescent patients. Although it can be a difficult task, it is vital to attempt to distinguish between different etiologies of pre-syncope and syncope and to know when further workup and evaluation are indicated. Obtaining a detailed history about the circumstances of the event is the most useful way to determine whether further workup is required. Typically, an ECG is required in the evaluation and many times it is the only test required.[23] Red flags for cardiac-related syncope are syncope with exertion or exercise, a lack of prodromal symptoms before the syncope, other associated cardiac symptoms, head or body injury at the time of syncope, and abnormal examination or ECG findings. Even if the baseline ECG is normal, concerning syncopal episodes with exertion require further workup, often including echocardiogram, cardiac ambulatory monitor, exercise stress test, extensive family history, and in some instances CT angiogram and/or cardiac MRI (**Table 3**).

Palpitations

A positive screen for palpitations means that a patient can be experiencing rapid, irregular, or

Table 3
Common causes of cardiac and noncardiac pediatric syncope

Causes	Features
Cardiac syncope	
Structural	Occurs without warning
• Coronary artery anomalies	No pre-syncopal prodrome
• Severe great vessels outflow obstruction	Event occurred during physical exertion
• Hypertrophic cardiomyopathy	Severe chest pain
Arrhythmia	Palpitations
• Atrioventricular block	Syncopal episode leading to need for
• Long QT Syndrome	resuscitative measures
• Short QT Syndrome	
• Wolff–Parkinson–White syndrome	
• Catecholaminergic polymorphic ventricular tachycardia	
Myocardia dysfunction	
• Cardiomyopathy (dilated, restrictive)	
• Myocarditis	
Noncardiac syncope	
Vasovagal	Pre-syncopal prodrome of lightheadedness or visual changes is common. Can have frequent pre-syncope without loss of consciousness. Associated with abrupt positional changes. Loss of consciousness is often <1 min
Autonomic dysfunction/orthostatic hypotension	Associated with marked increase in heart rate without hypotension on assuming an upright position. More common in females 5.1. Pre-syncopal symptoms with rare syncope. Associated with chronic fatigue and other vague systemic symptoms
Seizure	Tonic-clonic movements, tongue biting, or incontinence can be seen. prolonged period of confusion or postictal state after the event
Non-epileptic seizures	Associated with occurring at in predictable situations or when certain observers are present. Often occur during times of stress or high emotions. Episodes can be prolonged with abnormal movements not typical of seizures with epileptiform neural activity. Frequently during adolescent years. Often not a conscious act, but can be. This is typically a diagnosis of exclusion

prominent-feeling heart beats. Often this can be attributed to sinus tachycardia; however, atrial or ventricular dysrhythmias need to be ruled out. Children will often describe their heart as "pounding," "racing," "fluttering," "starting and stopping," or "beeping." Palpitations can be associated with pain, dizziness, shortness of breath, diaphoresis, nausea or vomiting, or syncope. Palpitations with exercise raise the level of concern. Typically, patients require an ECG and exercise stress test if the symptoms occur with exercise. Sometimes cardiac event monitors and echocardiograms can be helpful.

History of viral upper respiratory tract infection (COVID-19, influenza, rhinovirus, and so forth)
Even before the emergence of the COVID-19 infection related to the SARS-CoV-2 virus, there was a concern for myocarditis and sports participation. The primary reason for this is that myocarditis is well known to be a cause of SCD in athletes. At the beginning of the pandemic, there was a significant concern that COVID-19 was going to cause increased rates of myocarditis and put athletes at increased risk of SCA or SCD. Fortunately, overtime, this has found to not be true and the risk of myocarditis associated with COVID-19 is very low.[24,25]

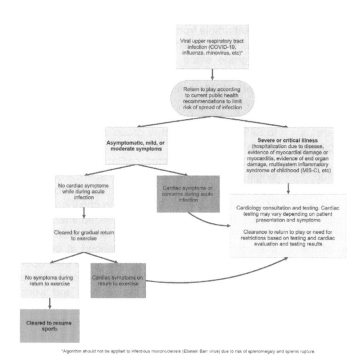

Fig. 3. Return to play algorithm after viral upper respiratory tract infection (COVID-19, influenza, rhinovirus, etc).

Owing to this, most patients can be cleared to return to sports after they have recovered from COVID-19 similar to the way they are cleared after other viral infection. Athletes with a history of myocardial injury or myocarditis or abnormal cardiac testing during an acute viral infection should have cardiac testing before participation. Athletes should also have a cardiac evaluation if they have cardiac symptoms during the acute illness or after returning to exercise (**Fig. 3**).

Family Medical History

Genetic heritability is an aspect of many diseases that confer an increased risk of SCD, such as cardiomyopathies, channelopathies, conduction abnormalities, and congenital heart disease to name a few. Providers will often find that the three family history questions in the AHA 14-point PPE need further explanation or examples to help patients give the most accurate history. Providing examples of sudden premature death (SIDS, unexplained drowning, or single-car accident of unknown cause) may aid in reducing ambiguity in the question. Many patients may be more comfortable using layman's terms, such as "enlarged heart" to represent cardiomyopathy. In other cases, patients and caregivers may be more familiar with interventions a family member may have had rather than a diagnosis. Asking about pacemaker insertion, implantable defibrillator devices, and heart transplant history can give clues about the underlying disease and whether it is applicable to the patient. This

is another case in which it is likely important to have a parent or caregiver available to supplement the history, as they may have more knowledge of the family's medical history than the patient.

How to Respond to an Abnormal Family History

When an athlete or family reports a positive family history of a cardiac disorder, efforts should be made to determine details regarding the exact diagnosis and whether or not genetic testing is available. These details will help guide the athlete's required evaluation and need for follow-up. Depending on the history, sports and exercise restriction may be required until details and cardiac testing is obtained.

Physical Examination

A detailed physical examination can uncover cardiovascular disease that may warrant further evaluation before sports participation clearance. The importance of vital signs, specifically blood pressure, should not be ignored. Elevated blood pressure is common. It can be a sign of underlying cardiac disease (eg, coarctation of the aorta) or undiagnosed hypertension and can predispose a patient to SCD/SCA. If a patient has upper extremity hypertension, careful attention should be paid to femoral pulses and blood pressure gradient between right arm and leg.

General examination is important to identify features that could be suspicious for certain syndromes. Providers should specifically physical stigmata of Marfan syndrome, such as abnormalities of spinal curvature, pectus deformities, hyperextensible joints, arm span to height ratio, myopia, and other characteristic facial features. The revised Ghent criteria can be used to determine the likelihood of Marfan syndrome or another connective tissue disorder. If there is any concern, then an echocardiogram is required to evaluate the aortic root, ascending aorta and mitral valve before sports participation.[19] Patients with findings consistent with Turner syndrome such as neck webbing, short stature, a low hairline, or low-set ears should also be evaluated with an echocardiogram given their risk of bicuspid aortic valve, coarctation of the aorta, and aortic aneurysms and dissections.

There should be a focus on identifying pathologic heart murmurs, abnormal or extra heart sounds, or rhythm irregularity. Benign murmurs are common in pediatrics, and it can be a challenge to differentiate between benign and pathologic. Benign murmurs typically are soft, systolic ejection murmurs that resolve with standing and do not radiate. Malignant murmurs are typically holosystolic, radiate to the back or neck, occur in diastole, or increase with standing.

Electrocardiogram Screening

There continues to be debate regarding whether or not ECGs should be added to the typical PPE. The European Society for Cardiology recommends including ECG for competitive athletes[26] and some countries mandate ECGs at various ages.[27–29] The most recent guidelines from the American College of Cardiology (ACC), AHA, and AMSSM suggest that ECG may be performed but did not recommend universal ECG screening.[19,30] There have been recent articles examining the utility of adding the ECG to the typical PPE.[31,32]

Advocates of ECG screening argue that the ECG is an inexpensive test, and with the use of new guidelines[33] and experienced interpreting physicians, the sensitivity and specificity are appropriate.[34]

Those who argue against ECG programs contend that resources should be focused elsewhere because ECGs have not been shown to save lives or prevent SCD, they add significant cost, and they lead to unnecessary, sometimes invasive, testing and procedures.

Interpretation of ECGs in pediatric patients can also be challenging. First, childhood ECGs are not as good at diagnosing cardiac pathology using typical standard criteria created for adults.

A recent article from Japan, where ECG screening has been mandated for all students in 1st, 7th, and 10th grade since 1973, demonstrated that the sensitivity of ECGs at diagnosing HCM using typical HCM criteria (pathologic Q waves, T-wave inversions, ST depression) was poor at 9% in first grade students. Sensitivity improved to 84% in the 7th grade group and 76% in 10th grade group.[35]

Second, as suggested earlier in this article, a single ECG in childhood or adolescence does not mean the patient will not develop an abnormal ECG or cardiac pathology later in childhood.

Last, the availability of experienced interpreting physicians may be limited. In general, pediatric primary providers are less experienced at ordering and interpreting ECGs compared with their adult counterparts. There are also significantly fewer pediatric cardiologists in the country and world compared with adult cardiologists.

Despite scientific evidence not being definitive, there will likely always be patient-led and family-led programs that offer ECG screening for pediatric and adolescent athletes. These programs should not be taken lightly and there should be significant thought into how the ECGs will be performed and interpreted as well as how abnormal results are communicated and further evaluated.

What Is Required If ECG Screening Is Pursued

1. Adequate training and experience of interpreting physicians
2. Appropriate privacy for performing of ECG and counseling (of patient and family) after ECG
3. An avenue for cardiologist evaluation and cardiac testing to be performed quickly and fully (ideally at the time of the screening, but if not, a few days later)

Other Nonroutine Modalities of Cardiac Evaluation

There have been studies evaluating the use of echocardiograms and exercise stress testing in PPEs. There has also been suggestion of using genetics[36] and [37] MRIs in preparticipation screening. These modalities certainly have advantages over the history, physical examination, and ECG, but given the cost and resources required for this type of testing and interpretation, widespread use of these modalities seems unlikely.

Return to the Cases

1. Adolescent with family history of HCM:

As the patient was 11 year old at the time of his initial normal cardiac evaluation, it was recommended

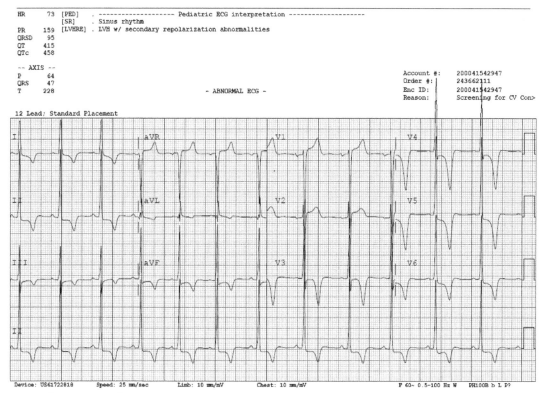

```
HR      73  [PED]   . -------------------- Pediatric ECG interpretation --------------------
            [SR]    . Sinus rhythm
PR     159  [LVHRE] . LVH w/ secondary repolarization abnormalities
QRSD    95
QT     415
QTc    458

-- AXIS --
P       64                                                          Account #:    200041542947
QRS     47                                                          Order #:      243662111
T      228                           - ABNORMAL ECG -               Enc ID:       200041542947
                                                                    Reason:       Screening for CV Con>

12 Lead; Standard Placement
```

Device: US61722818   Speed: 25 mm/sec   Limb: 10 mm/mV   Chest: 10 mm/mV   F 60~ 0.5-100 Hz W   PH100B b L P?

Fig. 4. Follow-up ECG of a now 15-year-old boy from Case 1 with a family history of HCM. This ECG is notable for voltage criteria for left ventricular hypertrophy and T-wave inversion in the inferolateral limb leads.

that he return to clinic in 4 years for repeat evaluation. At that visit, he reports that he has been participating in competitive sports without problems and has no cardiac symptoms. He has a normal physical examination with murmurs. His routine ECG (**Fig. 4**) shows left ventricular hypertrophy and significant

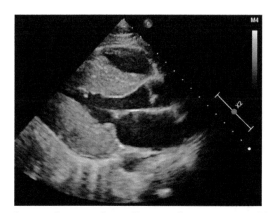

Fig. 5. Follow-up echocardiogram of a now 15-year old boy from Case 1 with a family history of HCM. This is a parasternal long axis image in 2D showing significant left ventricular hypertrophy and interventricular septal thickening to (1.6 cm, Z-score = 6.0), consistent with a diagnosis of hypertrophic cardiomyopathy).

T-wave inversions throughout the inferolateral leads (significantly different compared with initial ECG at 11 years of age, **Fig. 1**). His echocardiogram (**Fig. 5**) shows significant concentric hypertrophy of the left ventricle (ventricular septal thickness of 16 mm) and dynamic flow acceleration in the left ventricular outflow tract consistent with the diagnosis of HCM. This case highlights the importance of repeated screening in the pediatric population.

2. School-age child with an episode of syncope:

The 10-year-old patient with syncope underwent further cardiac evaluation due to the history of atypical nature of the syncope and the association with exercise. An ECG (**Fig. 6**) is notable for a correct QT duration of 597 ms. Laboratory testing does not reveal a secondary cause of prolonged QT interval. There is no family history of LQTS or other dysrhythmia. His routine echocardiogram is normal. The patient will be started on a beta blocker to reduce the risk of cardiac events and genetic testing demonstrated a pathogenic mutation in the KCNQ1 gene, which is associated with LQTS type 1. This case emphasizes the need to seriously consider all suspicious exercise-related events or symptoms, especially in school-age children who may not be able to communicate their

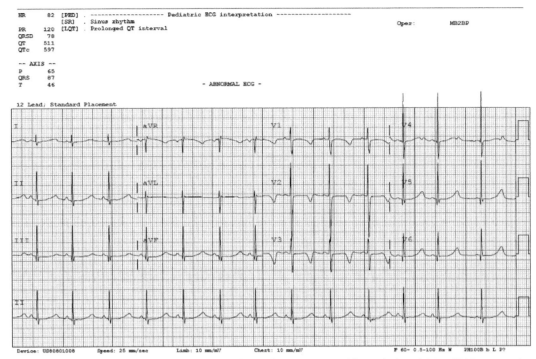

```
HR      82  [PED] . -------------------- Pediatric ECG interpretation --------------------
            [SR]  . Sinus rhythm                                                      Oper:        MB2BP
PR     120  [LQT] . Prolonged QT interval
QRSD    78
QT     511
QTc    597

-- AXIS --
P       65
QRS     87                           - ABNORMAL ECG -
T       46

12 Lead; Standard Placement

I           aVR          V1          V4

II          aVL          V2          V5

III         aVF          V3          V6

II

Device: U280801008   Speed: 25 mm/sec   Limb: 10 mm/mV   Chest: 10 mm/mV          F 60~ 0.5-100 Hz W   PH100B b L P?
```

Fig. 6. ECG from patient in Case 2 showing a prolonged QT segment with a calculated QTc of 597 ms, consistent with a diagnosis of LQTS.

symptoms as well. Syncope during exertion should always raise concern for cardiac pathology.

3. A collegiate baseball player with a history of KD:

As most patients with KD do not have significant residual coronary artery pathology, they do not require long-term antiplatelet or anticoagulation. The fact that the athlete remains on aspirin and dipyridamole should be a sign that he has residual coronary artery pathology and review of his past medical records and possible repeat cardiac testing is required before "clearance." On further review of this patient's history, it is determined that he was diagnosed with KD at the age of 3 years and at that time he had large coronary artery aneurysms. The coronary aneurysms have subsequently decreased in size to medium-sized coronary artery aneurysms (**Fig. 7**). The persistent aneurysms place him at risk for thrombus, so he has continued antiplatelet therapy.[21] Persistent coronary aneurysms related to KD require cardiology follow-up every 6 to 12 months and regular stress testing for inducible myocardial ischemia, both of which should be normal before sports clearance. As this patient enters adulthood, he should be considered for cardiac MRI to monitor for function and signs of ischemia and CT angiogram to monitor for coronary artery stenosis and calcification. This athlete has had those tests and they have been reassuring without evidence of inducible ischemia. The most recent ACC/AHA guidelines[19] allow him to participate in low to moderate static and dynamic competitive sports because he has no evidence of inducible ischemia.

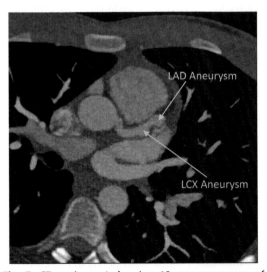

Fig. 7. CT angiogram showing 10 mm aneurysms of both the left anterior descending (LAD) and left circumflex (LCX) coronary arteries in a 15-year-old boy with a history of Kawasaki disease (KD).

Baseball is not a collision sport so there should be no restrictions related to his antiplatelet medications.

SUMMARY

While imperfect, the current sports preparticipation examination guidelines provide a solid framework for ensuring the safe engagement in physical activity for teenagers and children. It is also an important piece of health surveillance and maintenance in the pediatric population. As pediatric patients grow and develop quickly, so too does the need to regularly evaluate their health needs and risks. Informed and appropriately applied principles of the sports PPE will help providers give their patients the ability to be physically active with confidence.

CLINICS CARE POINTS

- Cardiac disease can present differently in children than in adults.
- Careful family history and symptom history is important when clearing pediatric patients prior to sports paticipation.
- Cardiac symptoms with exercise or exertion should have cardiac testing prior to participation.
- Exact type of testing should should be driven by patient symptoms.

DISCLOSURES

The authors have no relevant commercial or financial conflicts of interest in producing this article.

REFERENCES

1. Erickson CC, Salerno JC, Berger S, et al. Sudden death in the young: Information for the primary care provider. Pediatrics 2021;148(1). https://doi.org/10.1542/peds.2021-052044.
2. LaBotz M, Bernhardt DT. Preparticipation physical examination: is it time to stop doing the sports physical? Br J Sports Med 2017;51(3):152.
3. Gajewski KK, Saul JP. Sudden cardiac death in children and adolescents (excluding Sudden Infant Death Syndrome). Ann Pediatr Cardiol 2010;3(2):107–12.
4. Katritsis DG, Gersh BJ, Camm AJ. A clinical perspective on sudden cardiac death. Arrhythmia Electrophysiol Rev 2016;5(3):177–82.
5. Harmon KG, Asif IM, Maleszewski JJ, et al. Incidence, cause, and Comparative frequency of sudden cardiac death in National collegiate athletic association athletes: a decade in review. Circulation 2015;132(1):10–9.
6. Burns KM, Cottengim C, Dykstra H, et al. Epidemiology of sudden death in a population-based study of infants and children. J Pediatr X 2020;2. https://doi.org/10.1016/j.ympdx.2020.100023.
7. Winkel BG, Risgaard B, Sadjadieh G, et al. Sudden cardiac death in children (1-18 years): symptoms and causes of death in a nationwide setting. Eur Heart J 2014;35(13):868–75.
8. Maron BJ, Doerer JJ, Haas TS, et al. Sudden deaths in young competitive athletes analysis of 1866 deaths in the United States, 1980-2006. Circulation 2009;119(8):1085–92.
9. Maron BJ, Seidman JG, Seidman CE. Proposal for contemporary screening strategies in families with hypertrophic cardiomyopathy. J Am Coll Cardiol 2004;44(11):2125–32.
10. Faivre L, Masurel-Paulet A, Collod-Béroud G, et al. Clinical and molecular study of 320 children with Marfan syndrome and related type I fibrillinopathies in a Series of 1009 probands with pathogenic *FBN1* mutations. Pediatrics 2009;123(1):391–8.
11. Faivre L, Collod-Beroud G, Child A, et al. Contribution of molecular analyses in diagnosing Marfan syndrome and type I fibrillinopathies: an international study of 1009 probands. J Med Genet 2008;45(6):384–90.
12. Corrado D, Fontaine G, Marcus FI, et al. Arrhythmogenic right ventricular Dysplasia/cardiomyopathy. Circulation 2000;101(11). https://doi.org/10.1161/01.CIR.101.11.e101.
13. te Riele ASJM, James CA, Sawant AC, et al. Arrhythmogenic right ventricular Dysplasia/cardiomyopathy in the pediatric population. JACC: Clin Electrophysiol 2015;1(6):551–60.
14. DeWitt ES, Chandler SF, Hylind RJ, et al. Phenotypic Manifestations of arrhythmogenic cardiomyopathy in children and adolescents. J Am Coll Cardiol 2019;74(3):346–58.
15. Steinmetz M, Krause U, Lauerer P, et al. Diagnosing ARVC in pediatric patients Applying the revised task Force criteria: importance of imaging, 12-lead ECG, and genetics. Pediatr Cardiol 2018;39(6). https://doi.org/10.1007/s00246-018-1875-y.
16. Etoom Y, Govindapillai S, Hamilton R, et al. Importance of CMR within the task Force criteria for the diagnosis of ARVC in children and adolescents. J Am Coll Cardiol 2015;65(10):987–95.
17. Malhotra A, Dhutia H, Finocchiaro G, et al. Outcomes of cardiac screening in adolescent soccer players. N Engl J Med 2018;379(6):524–34.
18. Miller SM, Peterson AR. The sports preparticipation evaluation practice gaps. Available at: http://pedsinreview.aappublications.org/.

19. Maron BJ, Zipes DP, Kovacs RJ. Eligibility and Disqualification recommendations for competitive athletes with cardiovascular abnormalities: Preamble, principles, and general considerations. Available at: http://www.elsevier.com/about/.

20. Carek PJ, Futrell M, Hueston WJ. The preparticipation physical examination history: who has the correct answers? Clin J Sport Med 1999;9(3). https://doi.org/10.1097/00042752-199907000-00002.

21. McCrindle BW, Rowley AH, Newburger JW, et al. Diagnosis, treatment, and long-term Management of Kawasaki disease: a scientific statement for health professionals from the American heart association. Circulation 2017;135(17):e927–99.

22. Barbut G, Needleman JP. Pediatric chest pain Education gaps. Available at: http://pedsinreview.aappublications.org/.

23. Cannon B, Wackel P. Syncope Educational Gap. Available at: http://pedsinreview.aappublications.org/.

24. Martinez MW, Tucker AM, Bloom OJ, et al. Prevalence of inflammatory heart disease among professional athletes with prior COVID-19 infection who received systematic return-to-play cardiac screening. JAMA Cardiol 2021;6(7):745–52.

25. Moulson N, Petek BJ, Drezner JA, et al. SARS-CoV-2 cardiac Involvement in young competitive athletes. Circulation 2021;144(4):256–66.

26. Corrado D, Pelliccia A, Bjørnstad HH, et al. Cardiovascular pre-participation screening of young competitive athletes for prevention of sudden death: proposal for a common European protocol. Consensus statement of the study group of sport cardiology of the working group of cardiac Rehabilitation and exercise Physiology and the working group of myocardial and Pericardial diseases of the European Society of cardiology. Eur Heart J 2005;26(5). https://doi.org/10.1093/eurheartj/ehi108.

27. Corrado D, Basso C, Pavei A, et al. Trends in sudden cardiovascular death in young competitive athletes after implementation of a preparticipation screening program. JAMA 2006;296(13). https://doi.org/10.1001/jama.296.13.1593.

28. Steinvil A, Chundadze T, Zeltser D, et al. Mandatory electrocardiographic screening of athletes to reduce their risk for sudden death: Proven fact or wishful thinking? J Am Coll Cardiol 2011;57(11):1291–6.

29. HANEDA N, MORI C, NISHIO T, et al. Heart diseases discovered by mass screening in the schools of Shimane prefecture over a period of 5 years. Jpn Circ J 1986;50(12). https://doi.org/10.1253/jcj.50.1325.

30. Drezner JA, O'Connor FG, Harmon KG, et al. AMSSM position statement on cardiovascular pre-participation screening in athletes: current evidence, knowledge gaps, recommendations and future directions. Br J Sports Med 2017;51(3):153–67.

31. Petek BJ, Baggish AL. Current controversies in pre-participation cardiovascular screening for young competitive athletes. Expert Rev Cardiovasc Ther 2020;18(7):435–42.

32. Orchard JJ, Neubeck L, Orchard JW, et al. ECG-based cardiac screening programs: Legal, ethical, and logistical considerations. Heart Rhythm 2019;16(10):1584–91.

33. Sharma S, Drezner JA, Baggish A, et al. International recommendations for electrocardiographic interpretation in athletes. Eur Heart J 2018;39(16). https://doi.org/10.1093/eurheartj/ehw631.

34. Harmon KG, Zigman M, Drezner JA. The effectiveness of screening history, physical exam, and ECG to detect potentially lethal cardiac disorders in athletes: a systematic review/meta-analysis. J Electrocardiol 2015;48(3):329–38.

35. Yoshinaga M, Horigome H, Ayusawa M, et al. Electrocardiographic diagnosis of hypertrophic cardiomyopathy in the pre- and Post-diagnostic phases in children and adolescents. Circ J 2021. https://doi.org/10.1253/circj.CJ-21-0376. CJ-21-0376.

36. Magavern EF, Badalato L, Finocchiaro G, et al. Ethical considerations for genetic testing in the context of mandated cardiac screening before athletic participation. Genet Med 2017;19(5):493–5.

37. Angelini P, Muthupillai R, Lopez A, et al. Young athletes: Preventing sudden death by adopting a modern screening approach? A critical review and the opening of a debate. Int J Cardiol Heart Vasc 2021;34:100790.

Hypertension in Athletes
Clinical Implications and Management Strategies

Jason V. Tso, MD[a], Jonathan H. Kim, MD, MSc[b],*

KEYWORDS

• Hypertension • Cardiovascular risk • Athletes • Exercise

KEY POINTS

- Although habitual aerobic exercise lowers blood pressure, hypertension remains the leading cardiovascular disease in athletes and requires special considerations in this population.
- Sport-associated behaviors may predispose certain athletes to hypertension.
- Athletes with large body size and those engaged in primary strength training may be at increased risk of hypertension.
- Side-effect profiles and sport-specific legality must be considered when selecting pharmacotherapy for treatment of hypertension in athletes.

INTRODUCTION

Hypertension is an established and leading cause of cardiovascular (CV) morbidity and mortality in the United States.[1] Although athletes are generally viewed as paragons of health, hypertension is prevalent among youthful individuals, including athletes,[2,3] and associated with adverse outcomes in later-life.[4] In contrast to the general population, athletes present unique risk profiles that must be considered, such as deliberate weight gain in certain sports, strenuous isometric training regimens, supplement and stimulant use, and potential abuse of performance-enhancing agents. Moreover, intolerance of certain antihypertensive medications and avoidance of banned pharmaceuticals[5] must be considered in the evaluation and treatment of athletes with hypertension. In this review, we detail the epidemiology and clinical significance of elevated blood pressure (BP) in athletic populations, relationships with different training modalities, and special considerations for athletes, including BP assessment, tailored management strategies, and sports eligibility.

EPIDEMIOLOGY

Large-scale BP studies in athletes or highly active individuals are limited, although hypertension is generally accepted as the most prevalent CV risk factor present in athletes.[6] Routine BP assessment in younger athletes is generally limited to preparticipation physicals. Hypertensive BP at preparticipation physicals, according to the older Joint National Committee 7 (JNC-7) threshold of 140/90 mm Hg or greater, was 34.3% in a single center study of 2733 elite athletes.[2] Factors limiting the ascertainment of more precise hypertension prevalence estimates in athletes include significant heterogeneity in prior study designs, populations studied, and BP cutoff points used in prior studies. As such, hypertension prevalence among athletes has been reported from 0% to 83%.[7] However, in comparison to nonathletes,

Funding: Dr J.V. Tso has been supported by the Abraham J. & Phyllis Katz Foundation. Dr J.H. Kim is supported by the US National Institutes of Health/National Heart, Lung, and Blood Institute research grant K23 HL128795.
[a] Division of Cardiology, Emory University School of Medicine, 101 Woodruff Circle, WMB 319, Atlanta, GA 30322, USA; [b] Division of Cardiology, Emory Clinical Cardiovascular Research Institute, Emory University School of Medicine, 1462 Clifton Road, Northeast, Suite 502, Atlanta, GA 30322, USA
* Corresponding author.
E-mail address: jonathan.kim@emory.edu
Twitter: @jasontsomd (J.V.T.); @jonathankimmd (J.H.K.)

Cardiol Clin 41 (2023) 15–24
https://doi.org/10.1016/j.ccl.2022.08.002
0733-8651/23/© 2022 Elsevier Inc. All rights reserved.

hypertension is generally regarded as lower in prevalence in athletes.[6,7] With aging, as observed in the general population, the prevalence of hypertension in athletes increases.

It is well established that the presence of CV risk factors in young adults, particularly hypertension, is associated with later-life CV morbidity and mortality.[8–10] Independent of other established CV risk factors, the potency of increased BP on outcomes has been established, predicting incident atherosclerotic cardiovascular disease (ASCVD) and early, adverse CV outcomes.[11] Increases in afterload on the left ventricle (LV) also leads to the development of LV hypertrophy (LVH), typically with a concentric geometric remodeling pattern. Concentric LVH is also independently associated with incident heart failure, adverse CV outcomes, and increased mortality.[12] Relevant to physical performance, resting hypertension is associated with decreased exercise capacity.[13]

ARTERIAL STIFFNESS

Arterial stiffness is a critical mechanistic precursor to the development of hypertension.[14,15] Healthy arterial compliance provides a physiologic dampening effect that creates steady flow to end-organs and the microvasculature. Large artery stiffness (LAS) increases when this elastic reserve is lost, typically due to either aging or pathologic processes that lead to the deterioration of elastic tissues in the arterial walls.[14] Critically, increased LAS *precedes* systolic hypertension and likely contributes to maladaptive LV remodeling and dysfunction.[15] Increased pulsatility in the microvasculature because of LAS also contributes to end-organ injury, specifically in those that operate at low arteriolar resistance, such as the heart, kidney, and brain.[14] Aortic pulse wave velocity (PWV) is the clinical "gold" standard for assessing LAS and is independently associated with future CV events and mortality.[14,15]

Habitual aerobic exercise leads to improved LAS[16] but these benefits may not be present with strength/resistance training. In a small interventional study, Miyachi and colleagues prescribed an intense resistance training regimen to young men (N = 28) and noted decreased central arterial compliance and LAS after 4 months with compliance returning to baseline on detraining.[17] In a study comparing LAS between strength athletes (N = 14), endurance athletes (N = 14), and nonathlete controls (N = 7), Otsuki and colleagues found that endurance athletes had lower PWV than controls (thus more arterial compliance), whereas strength athletes had higher PWV and arterial stiffness compared with controls. Similar changes in

systemic arterial compliance (SAC) were present in endurance athletes with higher SAC observed versus the strength athletes. It is noteworthy that these differences were independent of BP.[18] These studies highlight the potential importance of sport-specificity in the context of vascular function given the suggestion of differential responses based on aerobic versus static exercise training regimens. In consideration of mechanisms underlying acquired hypertension in athletes, it remains uncertain if long-term strength and isometric training leads to the development of systemic hypertension.

ATHLETE-SPECIFIC BEHAVIORS

Coupled with pathophysiologic mechanisms underlying hypertension, several athlete-specific behaviors may predispose some athletes to hypertension and must be considered in the evaluation of an athlete with elevated BP measurements. Although causal associations remain elusive, these behavioral factors are common among many athletes based on sport-type and population. For example, weight lifters and American-style football (ASF) athletes typically must maintain high body weight and require high caloric intake with low-fiber diets.[19,20] Among Masters endurance athletes, generally defined as those over 35 years old, it is not uncommon for individuals to disclose unhealthy CV diets as regular high-doses of aerobic exercise allows for consumption of a calorie-dense, low-nutrition diet without increases in adiposity. Many Masters endurance athletes freely disclose sentiments of "eating whatever they want." Endurance athletes may also deliberately increase salt intake in an attempt to improve performance or prevent exercise-associated muscle cramping, a practice of questionable performance benefit.[21] Alcohol consumption may be increased in older endurance athletes, with one study of marathoners demonstrating higher BP and more alcohol intake compared to lower-performing athletes.[22] Finally, among competitive athletes, mental stress associated with chronic performance pressures may increase the risk of hypertension.[7]

For competitive athletes, body builders, and even some recreational weight lifters, abuse of illicit performance-enhancing drugs must be considered in the differential diagnosis of hypertension. Anabolic-androgenic steroids are associated with hypertension, accelerated ASCVD, and adverse cardiac remodeling.[23] Although banned in competitive sport, the global prevalence of anabolic steroid use has been estimated at 18.4% for recreational athletes and 13.4% for competitive athletes.[24] Legal substances also have considerable negative effects on BP. Caffeine, an ergogenic aid,[25] and other stimulants are commonly ingested by athletes across the age spectrum and in different sports during training and competition. Frequent use of unregulated energy drinks, which may be popular among younger athletes, can lead to arterial stiffening, hypertension, and exacerbation of underlying cardiac conditions.[26] In our experience, it is important to consider age and sport-type in assessing the likelihood of overused energy stimulants. In particular, in younger athletes, athletes engaged with more weight training, and baseball players who present with new hypertension, it is important to include a careful caffeine and energy drink intake as part of the clinical history. Finally, nonsteroidal anti-inflammatory drugs (NSAIDs) are commonly used as either prophylactic analgesics during training or to relieve injury-related pain.[27] Overused NSAIDs are associated with hypertension and have been implicated as a potential risk factor in high-collision sports such as American-style football.[28]

SPORT-TYPE

Sport-type is an important consideration in the risk of hypertension for athletes. Based on the most recent recommendations regarding sports eligibility and CV disease, sports are classified by the degree of peak dynamic and static load placed on the CV system during training or competition.[29] In general, athletic isometric disciplines are associated with hypertension.[7] In a systematic review of 51 athlete studies by Berge and colleagues, strength-trained athletes had higher BP than endurance-trained athletes (131.3 ± 5.3/ 77.3 ± 1.4 vs 118.6 ± 2.8/71.8 ± 1.2 mm Hg, $P < .05$).[7] The high body-mass index (BMI) of many strength athletes may increase the risk of hypertension. In a study of young professional Chinese strength athletes (N = 261) from Guo and colleagues, metabolic syndrome and dyslipidemia were common in athletes with high body weight, and athletes with the highest body weight had greater than 80% prevalence of hypertension using the 140/90 mm Hg or greater threshold.[30] Female athletes generally have lower BP than male athletes[31] but the association between increased body size and hypertension is present, regardless of sex.[32]

American-Style Football

Competitive ASF athletes have been extensively studied as a model of early hypertension and acquired CV risk.[33] Importantly, a high prevalence

of hypertension has been reported in both elite college and professional ASF athletes.[3,33–38] Weiner and colleagues conducted a longitudinal study of collegiate freshman ASF athletes and found that 47% of athletes had prehypertension and 14% had hypertension after one competitive season.[36] In a study of active professional ASF players, 13.8% had hypertension and 64.5% had prehypertension, significantly higher than a matched general population cohort.[38] Upon retirement, former professional ASF players maintain a hypertension prevalence of 37.8%, which is greater compared with the general population.[37] As the more lenient JNC-7 definitions were used for these older studies, hypertension prevalence is substantially higher using contemporary hypertension guidelines.[39] In a recent multicenter and longitudinal study across the collegiate ASF career using contemporary BP thresholds, 54% (32% stage 1%, 22% stage 2) of collegiate ASF athletes have hypertension before the initiation of the freshman season, which increases to 77% (33% stage 1%, 44% stage 2) by the conclusion of the junior season.[40] CV maladaptation occurs concomitant with increases in systolic BP (SBP) as longitudinal studies of collegiate ASF athletes have demonstrated an acquired maladaptive CV phenotype characterized by arterial stiffening,[41] hypertension,[36] impaired diastolic function,[34] impaired systolic function,[35,40] concentric ILVH,[3] and ventricular-arterial uncoupling[40] (**Table 1**).

Among ASF athletes, the lineman (LM) player position has been shown particularly at-risk for hypertension.[35,36,42] LM typically possess the highest BMI and SBP among all ASF athletes and experience a higher prevalence of sleep-disordered breathing, which has been correlated with arterial stiffening and diastolic dysfunction in ASF athletes.[43] Moreover, intentional weight gain and isolated static training, absent any aerobic exercise, are most notable among LM. Incident concentric LVH is associated with increased SBP among ASF athletes, with LM perhaps at greatest risk.[3,35,42] Among Olympic athletes, concentric LVH is rare but associated with hypertension, high BMI, and decreased exercise performance.[44] Similar to concentric LVH predicting increased CV risk in the general population,[12,45] the compilation of prior ASF data suggest that concentric LVH is not an adaptive form of cardiac hypertrophy and instead reflect emerging hypertension-related pathologic condition in athletes.

Masters Athletes

Hypertension in Masters athletes, although lower in prevalence compared with the general population, is still commonly encountered in clinical practice.[46] Numerous factors likely contribute to the overall lower burden, including lower BMI and habitual endurance training. Exercise and even early life physical activity confer beneficial BP effects in older athletes.[47] In a study from Laine and colleagues, former elite male athletes (N = 392; mean age 72.7 years; 17% endurance, 27% power, 56% mixed) had lower BP than nonathlete aged-matched controls.[48] This effect was most pronounced among former endurance athletes, indicating that previous high-volume dynamic activity may provide some degree of lasting protection from later-life acquired hypertension.

Masters endurance athletes, however, are not without CV risk and disease, including ASCVD. In a study from Mohlenkamp and colleagues, male marathon runners had more coronary artery calcification (CAC) than matched controls, with CAC further associated with myocardial late gadolinium enhancement.[49] Critically in this study, underlying CV risk in the athletes were driven by traditional CV risk with uncontrolled hyperlipidemia and a former-smoking prevalence of greater than 50%. Whether long-term ultraendurance exercise promotes the development of early coronary calcifications independent of traditional CV risk remains a controversial arena of study, with some data suggesting that some male Masters endurance athletes may harbor increased risk compared with nonathletic controls.[50,51] Merghani and colleagues studied low-risk Masters endurance athletes and found that cumulative training duration was independently associated with CAC greater than 70th percentile or greater than 50% coronary stenosis.[50] In general, underlying CV risk factors, including hypertension, are prevalent among Masters endurance athletes with ASCVD.[49,51]

THE EVALUATION OF ELEVATED BLOOD PRESSURE IN ATHLETES

Proper BP measurement can be challenging in athletes as infrequent medical contacts and nonstandard settings can lead to inaccurate assessment. Hastily taken BPs during high-stress preparticipation physicals may be the only annual medical contact for an athlete and can commonly lead to falsely elevated measurements. In accordance with contemporary ACC/AHA guidelines, standardized BP measurement should be performed to avoid these systematic errors.[39] Guidelines have also adjusted BP thresholds for hypertension from previous JNC-7 definitions. Stage 1 hypertension is now defined as SBP of 130 to 139 mm Hg or diastolic BP (DBP) of 80 to 89 mm Hg and stage 2 hypertension as SBP of

140 mm Hg or greater or DBP of 90 mmHg or greater.[39] Practitioners must remain cautious, recognizing which athletes may be at-risk for hypertension, such as ASF athletes[33] and carefully review risk factors that may predispose for hypertension. For all athletes with elevated BP readings, there must not be an assumption of a false-positive reading due to anxiety/stress levels, and at minimum, repeated measurements are necessary to affirm accurate BP measurements.[39]

Consistent with standardized BP measurements for all individuals, caffeine and exercise should be abstained for at least 30 minutes before measurement, and there should be 5 minutes of rest before BP measurement with the back supported, feet flat on the floor, and arm relaxed.[39] A properly sized cuff encompassing 80% of the arm should be used, which is relevant for strength athletes with large arm circumference and risk of falsely elevated readings. BP measurements should be averaged and assessed during multiple visits before establishing a diagnosis of hypertension.[39] An advantage for competitive athletes, particularly given many of these individuals are young and do not have access to home BP measurements, is the ability to obtain repeated measurements in the athletic training room. Ambulatory BP monitoring may be considered to confirm a diagnosis or evaluate for white coat hypertension, although clinical guidelines and outcome data are derived almost entirely from clinic BP measurement.[39,52]

For young athletes, a confirmed diagnosis of hypertension should be followed by a focused history and physical evaluating for secondary hypertension. The history should also include an extensive review of medications that can increase BP including NSAIDs and stimulants. Confidential discussions regarding performance-enhancing drugs should also be conducted, while acknowledging drug-testing results at the NCAA and professional levels will be available. The physical examination should include bilateral BP and pulse evaluation as an initial assessment for aortic coarctation,[53] abdominal auscultation to evaluate for renovascular hypertension, and evaluation of findings suggestive of corticosteroid excess.[52] Suspicion for secondary hypertension warrants comprehensive evaluation including renal ultrasound, obstructive sleep apnea screening, and testing for abnormal thyroid function and hyperaldosteronism.[54] Masters athletes should have additional laboratory tests including a lipid profile and diabetic screening for full ASCVD risk-stratification.[52]

All confirmed hypertensive athletes should receive a baseline electrocardiogram (ECG) and transthoracic echocardiogram. The ECG should

Table 1
Select studies of hypertension in American-Style football athletes

Study	Design	Key Findings
Tucker et al,[38] 2009	Cross-sectional study of 504 active professional ASF athletes vs 1959 men from the Coronary Artery Risk Development in Young Adults (CARDIA) study	• Hypertension[a] (13.8% [N = 67] vs 5.5% [N = 108], $P < .001$) and prehypertension (64.5% [N = 310] vs 24.2% [N = 473], $P < .001$) were more common in ASF athletes vs nonathletes
Weiner et al,[36] 2013	113 freshmen collegiate ASF athletes longitudinally studied during one competitive season	• SBP (116 ± 8 vs 125 ± 13 mm Hg, $P < .001$) and DBP (64 ± 8 vs 66 ± 10 mm Hg, $P < .001$) increased • 47% of athletes had prehypertension and 14% had hypertension[a] at postseason • ΔSBP was correlated with LVH in linemen
Lin et al,[35] 2016	30 linemen and 57 nonlinemen longitudinally studied during one competitive collegiate season	• SBP increased more in linemen than nonlinemen (Δ, 10 ± 8 vs 3 ± 7 mm Hg, $P < .001$) • 37% (N = 11) linemen developed LVH, of which 82% (N = 9) was concentric • Lineman position, postseason weight, SBP, LV wall thickness, and relative wall thickness predicted worse post-season GLS
Kim et al,[34] 2018	61 high school and 87 collegiate athletes longitudinally studied during one competitive season	• Only collegiate athletes demonstrated longitudinally increased SBP (131 ± 12–136 ± 12 mm Hg) and pulse-wave velocity (4.7 ± 0.7–5.0 ± 0.7 m/s) • Among collegiate athletes at postseason, SBP was associated with pulse-wave velocity and LV mass
Kim et al,[3] 2019	126 athletes studied during 3 y of collegiate ASF participation	• Athletes demonstrated increased weight (Δ, 4.74 kg, $P < .001$), SBP (Δ, 11.6 mm Hg, $P < .001$), and pulse-wave velocity (Δ, 0.24 m/s, $P = .007$) and decreased E′ (−1.7 cm/s, $P < .001$) • Increased SBP was associated with arterial stiffening ($\beta = 0.01$, $P = .007$) and concentric LVH (OR 1.04, $P = .02$)
Tso et al,[40] 2022	142 athletes analyzed during 3 y of collegiate ASF participation	• Hypertension[b] prevalence increased from 54% (22% stage 2) at baseline to 77% (44% stage 2) • Athletes demonstrated increased EA/ELV (Δ, 0.10, $P = .001$), indicating ventricular-arterial uncoupling • Increased SBP ($\beta = 0.029$, $P = .02$) and worsened GLS ($\beta = 0.045$, $P < .001$) predicted increased ΔEA/ELV

Abbreviations: ASF, American-style football, EA, arterial elastance; ELV, left ventricular end-systolic elastance; GLS, global longitudinal strain; LVH, left ventricular hypertrophy; SBP, systolic blood pressure.

[a] As defined by Joint National Committee 7 thresholds.
[b] As defined by 2017 American College of Cardiology/American Heart Association guidelines.

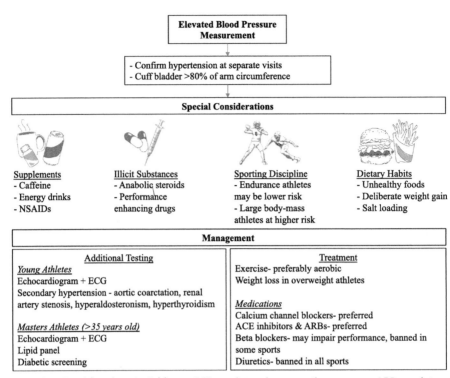

Fig. 1. Hypertension Considerations in Athletes. ACE, angiotensin-converting enzyme; ARB, angiotensin II receptor blocker; NSAIDs, non-steroidal anti-inflammatory drugs.

be interpreted by clinicians familiar with common athletic ECG findings.[55] Concentric LVH or LVH coupled with diastolic dysfunction should raise concern for hypertensive heart disease.[52,56] Adverse cardiac remodeling, when present, suggests longstanding hypertension warranting aggressive risk factor modification and treatment.

TREATMENT

Clinical treatment options for athletes include lifestyle modifications, education and counseling, and consideration of pharmacotherapy.(Fig. 1) Aerobic exercise regimens should be continued or encouraged in all athletes, particularly in primary strength athletes who are primarily committed to only static forms of training.[39] For athletes who require high body weight, such as ASF linemen, dietary patterns should be scrutinized, although acknowledging that high caloric intake is likely unavoidable during competitive sport training and participation. All hypertensive athletes should consider and reduce sodium intake and maintain high levels of dietary potassium, as both lead to favorable BP alterations.[39] Education and counseling the need to alter lifestyle habits on conclusion of the competitive sports career for later-life cardiac prevention is a critical

part of the management for athletes who must maintain high body weight.

Dietary change alone is often insufficient to reach target BP goals. Pharmacotherapy selection for athletes must include consideration of potential effects on performance and avoidance of drugs that are banned in sport. Angiotensin-converting enzyme inhibitors, angiotensin-receptor blockers, and dihydropyridine calcium channel blockers are generally considered first-line agents in athletic populations.[56] These drug classes are typically well tolerated with minimal side effects and are allowed by most governing sporting bodies.[5,57] Dihydropyridine calcium channel blockers may be preferred as they have no effect on heart rate and do not require monitoring of electrolytes or renal function. Beta-blockers may not be well tolerated or lead to reductions in aerobic performance and are also banned in sports dependent on limb stability and concentration (eg, golf and archery).[5] Nearly all diuretics, including thiazides, loop diuretics, and mineralocorticoid antagonists, are universally banned because they may mask other illicit substances.[5] Moreover, among recreational endurance athletes, concern for electrolyte and volume shifts with diuretics during endurance exercise may limit use in this population. Competitive athletes who require diuretics

Table 2
Athlete-specific considerations for antihypertensive medications

Medication Class	Selection in Athletes	Considerations
Dihydropyridine calcium channel blockers	Preferred	• First-line therapy in athletes • Well tolerated but may cause peripheral edema
ACE inhibitors and ARBs	Preferred	• First-line therapy in athletes • Well tolerated but may cause a nonproductive cough (more common with ACE inhibitors)
Nondihydropyridine calcium channel blockers	May be poorly tolerated	• Decreased chronotropy and inotropy, may reduce physical performance • Can be used to treat concomitant atrial fibrillation
Beta-blockers	Generally avoid in most athletes	• Decreased chronotropy and inotropy, may not be tolerated • Banned in precision sports (performance enhancer)
Diuretics and mineralocorticoid antagonists	Avoid in all competitive athletes	• Electrolyte shifts and volume depletion, may be poorly tolerated especially in endurance sports • Banned in all sports (weight loss and masking agent)

Abbreviations: ACE, angiotensin-converting enzyme, ARB, angiotensin receptor blocker.

require therapeutic-use exemptions to compete (**Table 2**).

SPORTS RESTRICTION AND RETURN-TO-PLAY

Athletes with essential hypertension are generally allowed to continue sports participation with no restrictions. However, with uncontrolled Stage 2 hypertension (SBP >160 mm Hg or DBP >100 mm Hg) or if signs of chronic end-organ damage are present, it is reasonable to restrict athletes from high static activities until BP control has been achieved.[52] Once BP is controlled, athletes should continue with regular BP surveillance on resumption of sport. Athletes with echocardiographic LVH and findings more suggestive of hypertension than exercise-induced cardiac remodeling do not need to be restricted from sport but require frequent BP reassessment to ensure that prompt and sustained BP control is attained.

EXERCISE BLOOD PRESSURE

During exercise, SBP normally increases 10 ± 2 mm Hg per metabolic equivalent as cardiac output increases with activity.[58] A portion of the population experiences a hypertensive response

to exercise (HRE), generally defined as an absolute SBP of 210 mm Hg or greater or increase of 60 mm Hg or greater in men or absolute SBP of 190 mm Hg or greater or increase of 50 mm Hg or greater in women during exercise testing.[58,59] HRE in those without resting hypertension predicts the development of future hypertension[60] and has been associated with carotid atherosclerosis[61] and increased risk of myocardial infarction.[62] These data, however, were obtained from observational studies of middle-aged individuals with established CV risk factors including smoking and hyperlipidemia. The clinical significance of HRE in younger and healthier athletes is unclear, and HRE in isolation does not require pharmacologic treatment in any population.

Experimental data linking HRE with CV pathologic condition in older athletes are limited. In a small study of 50 male marathon runners, runners with HRE had more CAC than those with a normal BP response to exercise (42.6 ± 67.8 vs 2.8 ± 6.0 Agatston units, $P = .036$).[63] In a porcine model of hypertension, Al-Mashadi and colleagues noted that local increases in pressure promoted infiltration of low-density lipoproteins in the coronary arteries.[64] This mechanism parallels increased coronary pressure in humans with HRE. Although the compilation of these small datasets are intriguing, studies investigating the association between HRE and cardiac pathologic condition in athletes are limited at this point, requiring more rigorous lines of future research.

CLINICAL UNCERTAINTIES

BP targets have been lowered in the latest ACC/AHA guidelines with more recent trials suggesting that even lower BP goals may further reduce CV risk.[65] This recurring question of "how low to go" with BP goals should also be applied to athletic populations, especially in athletes with CV risk factors. The compilation of longitudinal data in ASF cohorts suggest that early life hypertension leads to adverse CV remodeling that may contribute to adverse later-life CV outcomes.[3,36,40] Clinical trials of behavioral and pharmacologic intervention in young athletes with hypertension are warranted to determine whether early treatment may deter these maladaptive changes. Finally, examining the prevalence of hypertension in younger athletes as a function of sex, self-identified race, and other sport-types is a critical uncertainty that must be addressed in future studies.

SUMMARY

The evaluation and treatment of hypertension in athletes requires special considerations. Although habitual exercise training is protective against the development of hypertension, athletes are still at risk for hypertension and have additional unique considerations in the evaluation of hypertensive BPs. This is particularly relevant among strength-trained athletes, particularly those participating in ASF. In addition to ensuring athlete-specific risk factors are considered, pharmacologic treatment strategies must be carefully selected to avoid impaired athletic performance or using sport-specific banned drugs. Defining the range of hypertension prevalence in different populations of athletes, BP treatment goals, and the clinical significance of HRE represent evolving areas of research.

CLINICS CARE POINTS

- Among presumably healthy athletes, blood pressure evaluation requires careful attention and appropriate behavioral and pharmacologic treatment.

- Athletes with larger body size and predominantly strength-based training regimens, such as American-style football players, are at increased risk of hypertension.
- Athletes may not tolerate certain classes of blood pressure medications, and the legality of specific blood pressure medications in sport must be considered.

DISCLOSURE

Dr J.H. Kim receives compensation serving in his role as team cardiologist for the Atlanta Falcons. Dr J.V. Tso reports no disclosures.

FUNDING SOURCES

Abraham J & Phillis Katz Foundation from Dr J.V. Tso and the NIH/NHLBI for Dr J.H. Kim.

REFERENCES

1. Nambiar L, Lewinter MM, Vanburen PC, et al. Decade-long Temporal Trends in U.S. Hypertension-related cardiovascular mortality. J Am Coll Cardiol 2020;75(20):2644–6.
2. Hedman K, Moneghetti KJ, Christle JW, et al. Blood pressure in athletic preparticipation evaluation and the implication for cardiac remodelling. Heart 2019;105(16):1223–30.
3. Kim JH, Hollowed C, Liu C, et al. Weight gain, hypertension, and the emergence of a maladaptive cardiovascular phenotype Among US football players. JAMA Cardiol 2019;4(12):1221.
4. Yano Y, Reis JP, Colangelo LA, et al. Association of blood pressure Classification in young adults using the 2017 American college of Cardiology/American heart association blood pressure guideline with cardiovascular events later in life. JAMA 2018;320(17):1774.
5. World anti-Doping agency (WADA) Prohibited list. 2022. https://www.wada-ama.org/en/prohibited-list.
6. De Matos LD, Caldeira Nde A, Perlingeiro Pde S, et al. Cardiovascular risk and clinical factors in athletes: 10 Years of evaluation. Med Sci Sports Exerc 2011;43(6):943–50.
7. Berge HM, Isern CB, Berge E. Blood pressure and hypertension in athletes: a systematic review. Br J Sports Med 2015;49(11):716–23.
8. McCarron P, Smith GD, Okasha M, et al. Blood pressure in young adulthood and mortality from cardiovascular disease. Lancet 2000;355(9213):1430–1.
9. Pletcher MJ, Bibbins-Domingo K, Liu K, et al. Nonoptimal lipids commonly present in young adults and coronary calcium later in life: the CARDIA

(Coronary Artery Risk Development in Young Adults) study. Ann Intern Med 2010;153(3):137–46.

10. Baker JL, Olsen LW, Sørensen TIA. Childhood body-mass index and the risk of coronary heart disease in adulthood. N Eng J Med 2007;357(23):2329–37.

11. Whelton SP, McEvoy JW, Shaw L, et al. Association of normal systolic blood pressure level with cardiovascular disease in the absence of risk factors. JAMA Cardiol 2020;5(9):1011.

12. Drazner MH. The Progression of hypertensive heart disease. Circulation 2011;123(3):327–34.

13. Mazic S, Suzic Lazic J, Dekleva M, et al. The impact of elevated blood pressure on exercise capacity in elite athletes. Int J Cardiol 2015;180:171–7.

14. Chirinos JA, Segers P, Hughes T, et al. Large-artery stiffness in health and disease. J Am Coll Cardiol 2019;74(9):1237–63.

15. Kaess BM, Rong J, Larson MG, et al. Aortic stiffness, blood pressure Progression, and incident hypertension. JAMA 2012;308(9):875.

16. Bhuva AN, D'Silva A, Torlasco C, et al. Training for a first-Time marathon Reverses age-related aortic stiffening. J Am Coll Cardiol 2020;75(1):60–71.

17. Miyachi M, Kawano H, Sugawara J, et al. Unfavorable effects of resistance training on central arterial compliance. Circulation 2004;110(18):2858–63.

18. Otsuki T, Maeda S, Iemitsu M, et al. Relationship between arterial stiffness and athletic training Programs in young adult men. Am J Hypertens 2007;20(9):967–73.

19. Larson-Meyer DE, Krason RK, Meyer LM. Weight gain recommendations for athletes and Military Personnel: a critical review of the Evidence. Curr Nutr Rep 2022;11(2):225–39.

20. Jonnalagadda SS, Rosenbloom CA, Skinner R. Dietary practices, attitudes, and physiological status of collegiate freshman football players. J Strength Cond Res 2001;15(4):507–13.

21. McCubbin AJ, Cox GR, Costa RJS. Sodium intake Beliefs, Information Sources, and Intended practices of endurance athletes before and during exercise. Int J Sport Nutr Exerc Metab 2019;1–11.

22. Kim Y-J, Park Y, Kang D-H, et al. Excessive exercise habits in marathoners as Novel Indicators of masked hypertension. Biomed Res Int 2017;2017:1–7.

23. Baggish AL, Weiner RB, Kanayama G, et al. Cardiovascular Toxicity of illicit anabolic-androgenic steroid Use. Circulation 2017;135(21):1991–2002.

24. Sagoe D, Molde H, Andreassen CS, et al. The global epidemiology of anabolic-androgenic steroid use: a meta-analysis and meta-regression analysis. Ann Epidemiol 2014;24(5):383–98.

25. Pickering C, Grgic J. Caffeine and exercise: what Next? Sports Med 2019;49(7):1007–30.

26. Seifert SM, Schaechter JL, Hershorin ER, et al. Health effects of energy drinks on Children, Adolescents, and young adults. Pediatrics 2011;127(3):511–28.

27. Warden SJ. Prophylactic use of NSAIDs by athletes: a risk/benefit assessment. Phys Sportsmed 2010;38(1):132–8.

28. Tso J, Hollowed C, Liu C, et al. Nonsteroidal anti-inflammatory drugs and cardiovascular risk in American football. Med Sci Sports Exerc 2020;52(12):2522–8.

29. Levine BD, Baggish AL, Kovacs RJ, et al. Eligibility and Disqualification recommendations for competitive athletes with cardiovascular Abnormalities: Task Force 1: Classification of sports: dynamic, static, and impact: a Scientific Statement from the American heart association and American college of Cardiology. J Am Coll Cardiol 2015;66(21):2350–5.

30. Guo J, Zhang X, Wang L, et al. Prevalence of metabolic syndrome and its Components among Chinese professional athletes of strength sports with different body weight Categories. PLoS ONE 2013;8(11):e79758.

31. Pelliccia A, Adami PE, Quattrini F, et al. Are Olympic athletes free from cardiovascular diseases? Systematic investigation in 2352 participants from Athens 2004 to Sochi 2014. Br J Sports Med 2017;51(4):238–43.

32. Taha YK, Rambarat CA, Reifsteck F, et al. Blood pressure characteristics of collegiate female athletes: a call for more focused attention on young women's health. AHJ Plus 2022;13:100085.

33. Kim JH, Zafonte R, Pascuale-Leon A, et al. American-Style football and cardiovascular health. J Am Heart Assoc 2018;7(8):e008620.

34. Kim JH, Hollowed C, Patel K, et al. Temporal changes in cardiovascular remodeling associated with football participation. Med Sci Sports Exerc 2018;50(9):1892–8.

35. Lin J, Wang F, Weiner RB, et al. Blood pressure and LV remodeling among American-style football players. Jacc: Cardiovasc Imaging 2016;9(12):1367–76.

36. Weiner RB, Wang F, Isaacs SK, et al. Blood pressure and left ventricular hypertrophy during American-style football participation. Circulation 2013;128(5):524–31.

37. Albuquerque FN, Kuniyoshi FH, Calvin AD, et al. Sleep-disordered breathing, hypertension, and obesity in retired National Football League players. J Am Coll Cardiol 2010;56(17):1432–3.

38. Tucker AM, Vogel RA, Lincoln AE, et al. Prevalence of cardiovascular disease risk factors among National Football League players. JAMA 2009;301(20):2111–9.

39. Whelton PK, Carey RM, Aronow WS, et al. 2017 ACC/AHA/AAPA/ABC/ACPM/AGS/APhA/ASH/ASPC/NMA/PCNA guideline for the prevention, Detection, evaluation, and management of high blood pressure in adults: a report of the American

college of Cardiology/American heart association Task Force on clinical Pr. Hypertension 2018;71(6):e13–115.

40. Tso JV, Turner CG, Liu C, et al. Hypertension and ventricular–arterial uncoupling in collegiate American football athletes. J Am Heart Assoc 2022;11(6):e023430.

41. Kim JH, Sher S, Wang F, et al. Impact of American-style football participation on vascular function. Am J Cardiol 2015;115(2):262–7.

42. Tso JV, Turner CG, Liu C, et al. Association between race and maladaptive concentric left ventricular hypertrophy in American-style football athletes. Br J Sports Med 2022;56(3):151–7.

43. Kim JH, Hollowed C, Irwin-Weyant M, et al. Sleep-disordered breathing and cardiovascular Correlates in college football players. Am J Cardiol 2017;120(8):1410–5.

44. Caselli S, Cicconetti M, Niederseer D, et al. Left ventricular hypertrophy in athletes, a case-control analysis of interindividual variability. Int J Cardiol 2022;348:157–62.

45. Muiesan ML, Salvetti M, Monteduro C, et al. Left ventricular concentric Geometry during treatment adversely Affects cardiovascular Prognosis in hypertensive Patients. Hypertension 2004;43(4):731–8.

46. Shapero K, Deluca J, Contursi M, et al. Cardiovascular risk and disease among Masters endurance athletes: Insights from the Boston MASTER (Masters athletes Survey to evaluate risk) initiative. Sports Med - Open 2016;2(1).

47. Hernelahti M, Kujala UM, Kaprio J, et al. Hypertension in master endurance athletes. J Hypertens 1998;16(11):1573–7.

48. Laine MK, Kujala UM, Eriksson JG, et al. Former male elite athletes and risk of hypertension in later life. J Hypertens 2015;33(8):1549–54.

49. Mohlenkamp S, Lehmann N, Breuckmann F, et al. Running: the risk of coronary events : prevalence and prognostic relevance of coronary atherosclerosis in marathon runners. Eur Heart J 2008;29(15):1903–10.

50. Merghani A, Maestrini V, Rosmini S, et al. Prevalence of Subclinical coronary artery disease in Masters endurance athletes with a low atherosclerotic risk profile. Circulation 2017;136(2):126–37.

51. Aengevaeren VL, Mosterd A, Braber TL, et al. Relationship between Lifelong exercise volume and coronary atherosclerosis in athletes. Circulation 2017;136(2):138–48.

52. Black HR, Sica D, Ferdinand K, et al. Eligibility and Disqualification recommendations for competitive athletes with cardiovascular Abnormalities: Task Force 6: hypertension. Circulation 2015;132(22):e298–302.

53. Maron BJ, Friedman RA, Kligfield P, et al. Assessment of the 12-lead ECG as a screening test for Detection of cardiovascular disease in healthy general populations of young People (12–25 Years of age). Circulation 2014;130(15):1303–34.

54. Rimoldi SF, Scherrer U, Messerli FH. Secondary arterial hypertension: when, who, and how to screen? Eur Heart J 2014;35(19):1245–54.

55. Sharma S, Drezner JA, Baggish A, et al. International recommendations for Electrocardiographic Interpretation in athletes. J Am Coll Cardiol 2017;69(8):1057–75.

56. Martinez MW, Kim JH, Shah AB, et al. Exercise-induced cardiovascular Adaptations and Approach to exercise and cardiovascular disease: JACC State-of-the-Art review. J Am Coll Cardiol 2021;78(14):1453–70.

57. 2021-22 NCAA banned substances. In: National collegiate athletic association. 2021. https://www.ncaa.org/sports/2015/6/10/ncaa-banned-substances.aspx.

58. Sharman JE, Lagerche A. Exercise blood pressure: clinical relevance and correct measurement. J Hum Hypertens 2015;29(6):351–8.

59. Shim CY, Ha J-W, Park S, et al. Exaggerated blood pressure response to exercise is associated with Augmented rise of angiotensin II during exercise. J Am Coll Cardiol 2008;52(4):287–92.

60. Miyai N, Arita M, Morioka I, et al. Exercise BP response in subjects with high-normal BP: exaggerated blood pressure response to exercise and risk of future hypertension in subjects with high-normal blood pressure. J Am Coll Cardiol 2000;36(5):1626–31.

61. Jae SY, Fernhall B, Heffernan KS, et al. Exaggerated blood pressure response to exercise is associated with carotid atherosclerosis in apparently healthy men. J Hypertens 2006;24(5):881–7.

62. Laukkanen JA, Kurl S, Salonen R, et al. Systolic blood pressure during Recovery from exercise and the risk of Acute myocardial infarction in middle-aged men. Hypertension 2004;44(6):820–5.

63. Kim CH, Park Y, Chun MY, et al. Exercise-induced hypertension can increase the prevalence of coronary artery plaque among middle-aged male marathon runners. Medicine (Baltimore) 2020;99(17):e19911.

64. Al-Mashhadi RH, Al-Mashhadi AL, Nasr ZP, et al. Local pressure Drives low-density lipoprotein Accumulation and coronary atherosclerosis in hypertensive Minipigs. J Am Coll Cardiol 2021;77(5):575–89.

65. Zhang W, Zhang S, Deng Y, et al. Trial of intensive blood-pressure control in older Patients with hypertension. N Eng J Med 2021;385(14):1268–79.

The Acute Impact of Endurance Exercise on Right Ventricular Structure and Function
A Systematic Review and Meta-analysis

Tristan Ramcharan, MD[a,b], Jamie Edwards, MSc[c], Jamie O'Driscoll, PhD[c],*, Michael Papadakis, MD[d]

KEYWORDS

- Adaptation • Endurance • Ultraendurance • Exercise • Right ventricle

KEY POINTS

- Endurance exercise is associated with acute RV dilatation and reduction in systolic function.
- There is a dose–response relationship because acute RV effects seem to be amplified following ultraendurance events.
- Those training more hours per week demonstrate a larger acute reduction of RVFAC following endurance events.
- RV systolic impairment resolves within a week following acute exercise, suggesting a reversible, short-term impact.

INTRODUCTION

The benefits of regular exercise for cardiovascular health are well publicized, and at population level, evidence suggests that more exercise is better (**Fig. 1**).[1,2] Regular exercise is associated with several cardiac adaptations, which is collectively referred to as "the athlete's heart." Such adaptations are evident in those who participate in regular training and competitions in sports of moderate to high intensity and are more prevalent in individuals participating in endurance sports. Since 1979, there have been in excess of 50 studies that have investigated the effect of endurance exercise on the left ventricle (LV). Studies suggest acute impairment of LV systolic and diastolic function postendurance exercise with increased LV volume and mass in the long term.[1,3,4]

In recent years, attention has focused on the right heart, with suggestions that the right ventricle (RV) is exposed to disproportionately increased workload during exercise compared with the LV.[5] At rest, the RV functions against a very low resistance and highly compliant pulmonary circulation. However, during exercise, right ventricular wall stress increases 30-fold, reflecting a minimal reduction in pulmonary vascular resistance and a significant rise in pulmonary artery systolic pressures.[6] As such, there are significant hemodynamic changes that occur during endurance exercise, which may magnify during ultraendurance events, leading to acute RV insult and reduced function.[7] Some researchers have gone a step further and postulated an exercise-induced right ventricular arrhythmogenic cardiomyopathy model in endurance athletes caused

a Heart Unit, Birmingham Children's Hospital, Birmingham, United Kingdom; b MSc Sports Cardiology, St George's, University of London, London, United Kingdom; c School of Psychology and Life Sciences, Canterbury Christ Church University, Kent CT1 1QU, United Kingdom; d Cardiovascular Clinical Academic Group, St George's, University of London, London, United Kingdom
* Corresponding author.
E-mail address: jamie.odriscoll@canterbury.ac.uk

Cardiol Clin 41 (2023) 25–34
https://doi.org/10.1016/j.ccl.2022.08.004
0733-8651/23/© 2022 Elsevier Inc. All rights reserved.

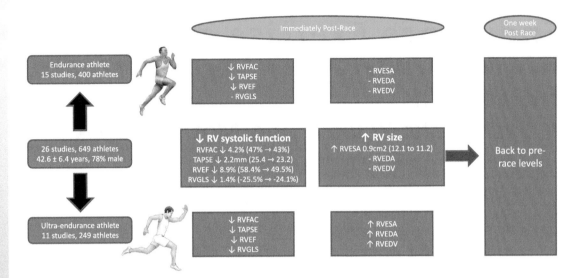

Fig. 1. Graphical abstract. RVEDA, right ventricular end-diastolic area; RVEDV, right ventricular end-diastolic volume; RVEF, right ventricular ejection fraction; RVESA, right ventricular end-systolic area; RVFAC, right ventricular fractional area change; RVGLS, right ventricular global longitudinal strain; TAPSE, tricuspid annular plane systolic excursion.

by cumulating RV insults and inadequate recovery time.[8,9]

To understand the acute impact of endurance exercise on RV structure, function, and mechanics, we performed a systematic review and meta-analysis. To explore a dose–response relationship between endurance exercise and acute RV changes, we further performed a subgroup analysis between endurance and ultraendurance events.

METHODS

This systematic review and meta-analysis was performed according to the PRISMA guidelines,[10] and is registered with PROSPERO (Reference: CRD42022302907). A systematic literature search was carried out using the Healthcare Databases Advanced Search (Embase, Medline, and PubMed) for articles published in English language only, using "((("right ventric*") AND (Endurance)) AND (Exercise)) AND (Athlete)." No restrictions or filters were applied to the search. Full-text articles were accessed from the St George's University Library catalog, NHS Open Athens, University of Birmingham catalog, and Clinical Key. Conference abstracts were also reviewed to gauge upcoming/unpublished research.

Following the exclusion of duplicates, articles were screened by title and then by abstract for relevance. Appropriate studies were then evaluated by full text according to the inclusion criteria of, "studies reporting acute impact of exercise on

the RV," "at least one pre-exercise and postexercise functional, structural, or mechanic RV parameter measurement," "endurance or ultraendurance sporting events," and "adult only studies." For this review, endurance exercise is defined as continuous exercise greater than 1.5 hours and ultraendurance as greater than 4 hours.[3,11] Following study recruitment, the respective premeans and postmeans, and standard deviations of all included studies were extracted. When data were reported in a different format (ie, standard error), they were appropriately converted.

Quantitative Analysis

The extracted raw data were manually inputted into the statistical analysis software Comprehensive Meta-Analysis version 3 (Biostat, Englewood, NJ). All data for each individual parameter were pooled and analyzed for weighted mean differences (WMD) with corresponding 95% confidence intervals (CI). Subgroup analysis of event type was performed to discern any differences in acute RV changes between endurance and ultraendurance events. Separately, where sufficient data were present, metaregression analyses were run to determine the effects of any potential moderators on acute RV changes. The moderators analyzed were age, sex, and training status. Statistical heterogeneity was assessed for each outcome via the I^2 statistic with a significance threshold of greater than 40%.[12] Once beyond this threshold, random effects analysis was selected.[12] Additionally, post hoc Egger tests were run to assess for potential publication bias by assessing the presence of funnel plot asymmetry.[13] The analysis of any given outcome was considered significant with $P < 0.05$ and a Z >2.

RESULTS
Characteristic of Included Studies

Full details of screened and included studies are seen in **Fig. 2**. Twenty-six studies[8-32] over a 32-year period were included (**Table 1**). In total, there were 649 athletes, with a mean age of 42.6 ± 6.4 years. Seventy-eight percent of all athletes were male. Of the 26 studies, 15 involved endurance events and 11 involved ultraendurance events. Imaging modalities used included a combination of transthoracic echocardiography (TTE) and cardiac MRI (CMR). All analyses were performed via a random-effects model because of significant heterogeneity.

Impact on Right Ventricle Systolic Function

There was a significant reduction in RV systolic function postexercise across studies (**Fig. 3**). Using traditional echocardiography markers, right ventricular fractional area change (RVFAC) was measured in 16 studies with a WMD reduction of 4.2% (95% CI, 1.8%–6.6%; I^2 = 97.3%; P = 0.001), from 47% before exercise to 43% postexercise. Tricuspid annular plane systolic excursion (TAPSE) was measured in 12 studies

and reduced by a WMD of 2.2 mm (95% CI, 0.5–3.9 mm; I^2 = 96.3%; P = 0.011), from 25.4 mm to 23.2 mm postexercise. Using three-dimensional TTE or CMR, right ventricular ejection fraction (RVEF) was measured in nine studies and was shown to be reduced by a WMD of 8.9% (95% CI, 2.8%–15%; I^2 = 99.2%; P = 0.004) from 58.4% to 49.5% following exercise. Using advanced longitudinal functional indices, right ventricular global longitudinal strain (RVGLS) was measured in nine studies and was shown to reduce by a WMD of 1.4% (95% CI, 0.6%–2.2%; I^2 = 93.0%; P = 0.001) from −25.5% to −24.1% following exercise. Right ventricular S′ and strain rate did not significantly differ pre-exercise and postexercise.

Seven studies[9,10,13,14,19,21] reassessed RV function following recovery from acute exercise, of which five showed normalization of all markers within 1 week.[9,10,13,19,21] The remaining two studies showed normalization of the RVFAC and TAPSE but persistent reduction of RV S′, although the WMD was not reduced.[14,19]

Comparing the studies reporting on ultraendurance events with endurance events, there was no significant difference in reduction of RVEF or RVFAC before and after exercise. However, there was a greater attenuation in RVGLS (less negative) following ultraendurance compared with endurance events (WMD, 2.2% vs 0.01%; P = 0.006) (**Fig. 4**). In fact, when analyzed separately, RVGLS

Fig. 2. PRISMA search methodology.

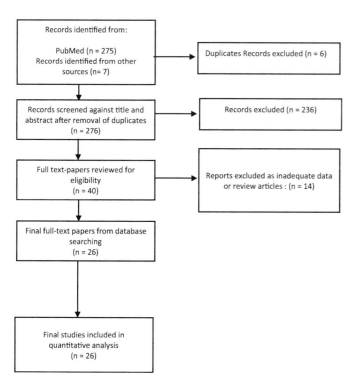

Table 1
Details of studies looking at acute endurance exercise effects

Study, Year	Country	Number of Participants	Male/Female Ratio	Mean Age, Years (SD)	Event
[a]Douglas et al,[22] 1990	United States	41	22:19	38 (10)	Ironman triathlon
[a]Carrio et al,[23] 1990	Spain	10	Unk	Unk	Ultramarathon
[a]Davila-Roman et al,[14] 1997	United States	14	Unk	Unk	High-altitude ultramarathon
Neilan et al,[24] 2006	United States	20	10:10	34 (10)	Marathon
Neilan et al,[25] 2006	United States	60	41:19	41 (11)	Marathon
Neilan et al,[26] 2006	United States	17	12:5	37	Rowers
Oxborough et al,[27] 2006	United Kingdom	35	29:6	30 (8)	Marathon
[a]La Gerche et al,[28] 2008	Australia	26	Unk	32	Ironman triathlon
Mousavi et al,[20] 2009	Canada	14	8:6	33 (6)	Marathon
Trivax et al,[29] 2010	United States	25	13:12	39 (9)	Marathon
O'Hanlon et al,[30] 2010	United Kingdom	17	17:0	34 (7)	Marathon
[a]Oxborough et al,[31] 2011	United Kingdom	16	12:4	42 (8)	Ultramarathon
Oomah et al,[32] 2011	Canada	15	7:8	32 (6)	Half-marathon
Karlstedt et al,[33] 2012	Canada	25	21:4	55 (4)	Marathon
Schattke et al,[34] 2012	Germany	21	21:0	46 (15)	Marathon
[a]La Gerche et al,[8] 2012	Australia	40	36:4	37 (8)	Ultratriathlon
Claessen et al,[35] 2014	Belgium	14	14:0	36 (6)	Cycling
[a]Lord et al,[36] 2015	United States	15	14:1	40 (8)	Ultramarathon
[a]Sanz de la Garza et al,[19] 2016	Spain	55	55:0	37 (7)	High-altitude ultramarathon
[a]Maufrais et al,[37] 2016	France	15	15:0	46 (13)	Ultramarathon
Stewart et al,[38] 2017	Australia	23	23:0	28 (8)	Cycling
Gajda et al,[39] 2019	Poland	12	7:5	Unk	Swimmers
Martinez et al,[40] 2019	Spain	33	26:7	41 (7)	Swimmers
[a]Christou et al,[41] 2020	Greece	25	19:8	45 (7)	Ultramarathon
[a]Coates et al,[42] 2020	Canada	8	6:2	45 (10)	Ultramarathon
Chen et al,[43] 2021	Germany	50	40:10	45 (10)	Triathlon

Abbreviations: SD, standard deviation; Unk, unknown.
[a] Ultraendurance events.

did not significantly change following an endurance event (WMD, 0.01%; 95% CI, -1.22% to +1.25%; $P = 0.987$; three studies), but was significantly depressed (less negative) following ultraendurance (WMD, 2.2%; 95% CI, + 1.26% to +3.14%; $P < 0.001$; six studies). There was insufficient data to compare TAPSE, RV S′ and right ventricular S′ and strain rate.

Impact on Right Ventricle Diastolic Function

RV diastolic function was assessed in five studies using Doppler imaging (E/A), myocardial tissue velocity (E′/A′), and/or strain imaging (SR E/A), but there were insufficient data to perform quantitative analyses.

Impact on Right Ventricle Size

Change in RV size was assessed by using either RV area or volume, using TTE or CMR. Only right ventricular end-systolic area (RVESA), which was measured in 12 studies, showed an increase by a WMD of 0.9 cm2 (95% CI, 0.1–1.7 cm2; $I^2 = 96.9\%$; $P = 0.028$) from 11.2 cm2 to 12.1 cm^2 following exercise. There were insufficient study data to perform quantitative analysis for right ventricular end-systolic volume. Both right

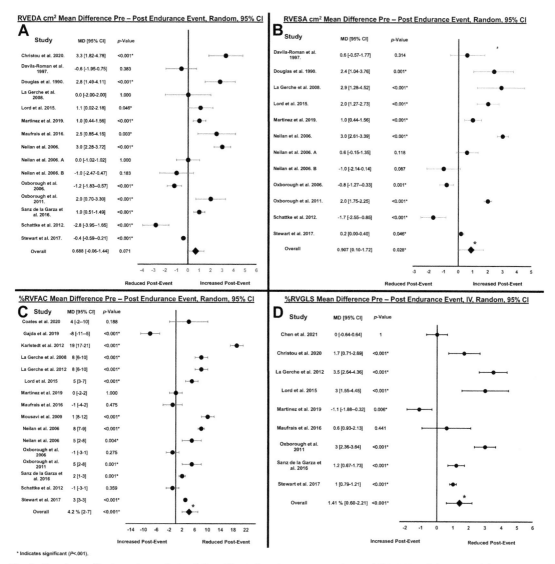

Fig. 3. Random-effects meta-analysis of the effect of endurance exercise on (*A*) RVEDA, (*B*) RVESA, (*C*) RVFAC, and (*D*) RVGLS. MD, mean difference.

ventricular end-diastolic area (RVEDA: WMD of 0.7 cm^2; 95% CI, -0.1 to 1.4 cm^2; I^2 = 93.3%; P = 0.071) and right ventricular end-diastolic volume (RVEDV: WMD of 19.97 mL; 95% CI, -11.4 to 51.3 mL; I^2 – 99.1%; P = 0.21) showed an increase, which, however, did not achieve significance.

Davila-Roman and colleagues[14] reported normalization in RV size after 24 hours of recovery following the endurance exercise.

Comparing ultraendurance with endurance events demonstrated that increase in RVEDA was significantly greater following ultraendurance compared with endurance events (WMD, 1.5 vs −0.1 cm2; P = 0.017; see **Fig. 4**). When analyzed

separately, RVEDA did not change following endurance events (WMD, −0.1 cm^2; 95% CI, -1.2 to −0.9 cm^2; P = 0.791; seven studies), whereas it was significantly increased following ultraendurance events (WMD, 1.5 cm^2; 95% CI, 0.5 to 2.5 cm^2; P < 0.001; eight studies). Similarly, change in RVESA was greater following ultraendurance compared with endurance events (WMD, 1.9 vs 0.2 cm^2; P = 0.006; see **Fig. 4**), and when analyzed separately, RVESA did not change following endurance events (WMD, 0.2 cm^2; 95% CI, -0.8 to 1.2 cm^2; P = 0.699; seven studies), but significantly increased following ultraendurance events (WMD, 2 cm^2; 95% CI, 0.7–

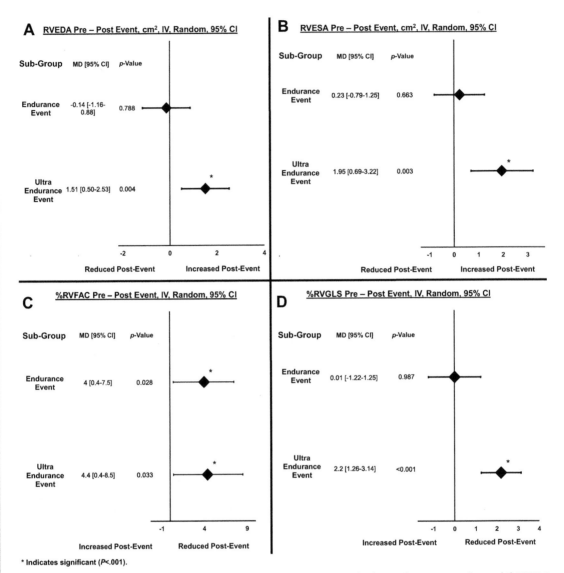

Fig. 4. Random-effects meta-analysis comparing endurance exercise with ultraendurance exercise on (A) RVEDA, (B) RVESA, (C) RVFAC, and (D) RVGLS.

3.2 cm²; *P* = 0.003; 5 studies). There were insufficient data to compare RVEDV.

Impact on Right Ventricle Pressure

Tricuspid regurgitant velocity is used to estimate right ventricular systolic pressure (RVSP), which in the absence of right ventricular outflow tract obstruction, approximates pulmonary artery systolic pressure (PASP). Five studies assessed change in RVSP/PASP following acute endurance exercise. No significant increase in pressure was noted (WMD, 2.0 mm Hg; 95% CI, -13.1 to 9.1 mm Hg; *I*² = – 99.5%; *P* = 0.72).

Moderator Analyses and Publication Bias

Moderator analyses were run to assess the effects of age, sex, and training status on any of the functional or structural RV changes. There was no significant moderator effect of age or sex. Conversely, moderator analysis of training status demonstrated a significant association with RVFAC, with those training more hours per week demonstrating a larger acute reduction following endurance events (*b* = 0.0072; *P* < 0.001). RVEDA showed no significant effect from training status, whereas there were insufficient data for analysis for RVEF, RVGLS, RVEDV, right ventricular end-systolic volume, and RVESA.

RVEF ($P = 0.037$) was the only parameter to produce statistically significant funnel plot asymmetry on the Egger regression test, indicating publication bias.

DISCUSSION

Our meta-analysis suggests a transient increase in RV size with associated reduction of the systolic function after acute endurance exercise. These effects seem to be more pronounced with ultraendurance events and reverse within a week.

Acute Impact of Endurance Exercise on the Right Ventricle

The most consistent finding across individual studies and a previously published meta-analysis is the acute reduction of RV systolic function postendurance events, as evident by several echocardiographic and CMR indices. Although it is difficult to determine cause and effect, individual studies suggest that it is the acute increase in PASP and therefore RV afterload during endurance exercise, that most likely accounts for the acute RV dysfunction. The thick walls of the LV and the ability of the systemic circulation to reduce vascular resistance, results in proportionately lower increase in the systolic blood pressure and LV "wall stress." The RV is a thin-walled structure that normally contracts against a low-pressure circulation. During exercise it must considerably increase its cardiac output to match the LV cardiac output.[15] Given the limited ability of the pulmonary vascular resistance to reduce further, the increased cardiac output results in an increase in PASP, which corelates with exercise intensity, with values of up to 90 mm Hg recorded in elite endurance athletes.[16,17] The higher the RV afterload, the greater the RV "wall stress." Consequently, the RV is disproportionally impacted by endurance exercise, leading to acute impairment in ventricular contractility, which recovers once RVSP/PASP normalizes. Indeed, our meta-analysis did not identify persistently elevated RVSP/PASP postevent suggesting that it is the repeated transient elevations in RV pressures and RV afterload that are likely to be responsible for the acute and the reported chronic RV changes.

Alternately, as the RV dilates, less "contraction" is needed to produce similar stroke volume, and this could partly explain the reduction in systolic function. Lord and colleagues[18] used area-deformation loops to suggest that this RV dilation with reduced systolic function may be a form of adaptation and not dysfunction. However, this contrasts with some chronic endurance athletes having resting RV dilation but without systolic impairment.

The Importance of Exercise Duration

This meta-analysis demonstrates that the significant reduction in RV systolic function following acute endurance exercise is amplified following ultraendurance events, giving weight to a dose–response relationship between exercise duration and acute systolic RV functional impairment.[19,22] The acute RV functional impairment reported transcends global and longitudinal function. The RVGLS is attenuated in a dose–response manner with increasing endurance exercise, suggesting that the RV functional impairment is not simply a hemodynamic effect from fluid shifts, but that endurance exercise has a real effect on the RV myocardium.

The meta-analysis also shows the increase in RV size following acute endurance exercise is amplified following ultraendurance events. Sanz de la Garza and colleagues[19] showed that RV dilation is proportional to the duration and intensity of exercise with a similar dose–response relationship to systolic function. Studies that examined RV size following recovery from acute endurance events showed normalization to pre-event size.[14] Similarly, studies of chronic adaptation to exercise show significant RV enlargement in endurance athletes compared with sedentary control subjects, suggesting that endurance exercise has acute temporary and chronic effects on RV adaptation.

Clinical Implications

Clinicians should be aware of the transient increase in RV size and reduction in RV systolic function postendurance exercise and the incremental impact of ultraendurance events. This is relevant to physicians supervising endurance events but also to those who may encounter athletes following endurance events as part of cardiac screening or during acute presentation with cardiac or noncardiac symptoms. The presence of reduced RV systolic function with a dilated RV size should be interpreted in the right clinical context to avoid a cascade of potentially unnecessary further tests and erroneous diagnosis. This is even more important when one considers that the acute RV changes have also been associated with transient increase of serum troponin levels.[20]

The attenuated systolic function seems to resolve within a week following acute exercise, suggesting that the acute effect of endurance exercise has only a short-term impact on RV systolic function. The chronic repeated impact of endurance exercise on RV function and mechanics remains to be elucidated. The association of more training hours per week with greater acute reduction of RVFAC following endurance events offers some support to the suggestion that veteran endurance athletes can develop an acquired, exercise-induced arrhythmogenic right ventricular cardiomyopathy (ARVC) phenotype,[7,21] because of repeated insults from endurance events, when coupled with inadequate recovery between events.

CRITIQUE OF LITERATURE
Strengths

This systematic review and meta-analysis has several strengths. These include an extensive review of the literature on the acute effects of endurance exercise on RV function and mechanics, with 26 articles and almost 650 athletes included. This allowed multiple parameters to be compared, with no studies having vastly different results increasing confidence in conclusions. Additionally, all studies were prospective and designed to allow postexercise investigations to be performed as close to activity completion as possible to improve accuracy in the findings.

A previous meta-analysis on the effect of endurance exercise on the RV by Elliott and Gerche[11] in 2014, using 14 studies, including some that have been reviewed in our study, also demonstrated an increase in RV size and decrease in RV function from endurance exercise. Our meta-analysis builds on this work, confirming the effect on RV size/function but also underlines the dose–response relationship of endurance exercise by comparing endurance with ultraendurance events.

Limitations

There are several limitations from individual study designs and from comparing studies with each other. First, studies included used predominantly male populations, introducing sex bias and making subanalysis of sex differences less powered. As such the lack of any sex differences in our study should be interpreted with caution. Additionally, most studies did not mention ethnicity, making it difficult to comment on the effect of ethnicity on RV responses to exercise. Studies are heavily biased toward White, male endurance athletes and further work must improve the demographic and sex distribution of included athletes to better represent the realities of modern endurance sport so that one can apply research evidence more accurately into clinical practice. Potential publication bias should also be considered when interpreting RVEF. Finally, consideration of age in future studies would be a useful subanalysis, particularly to compare adolescent with veteran endurance athletes, and to explore whether the demonstrated changes in RV size and function are more pronounced in veteran athletes because of a potentially less compliant circulation.

SUMMARY

Acute endurance exercise results in RV dilation and attenuated systolic function, which is dose dependent, with greater attenuation as the volume of endurance exercise increases. These effects reverse within a week.

Future research is required to investigate the implications of these acute responses to chronic adaptions in athletes and further explore the influence of sex, ethnicity, and age.

CLINICS CARE POINTS

- Following acute endurance exercise, right ventricular size is increased while systolic function is impaired.
- Post-exercise changes in the right ventricle are dose-dependent with the largest effects seen following ultra-endurance events.
- These right ventricular changes should reverse, returning to baseline within 1 week.

DISCLOSURE

M. Papadakis has received funding from the charitable organization Cardiac Risk in the Young, which supports cardiac screening of young and athletic individuals.

REFERENCES

1. Middleton N, Shave R, George K, et al. Left ventricular function immediately following prolonged exercise: a meta-analysis. Med Sci Sports Exerc 2006; 38(4):681–7.
2. Loef M, Walach H. The combined effects of healthy lifestyle behaviors on all-cause mortality: a systematic review and meta-analysis. Prev Med 2012; 55(3):163–70.
3. Lord R, Oxborough D, Somauroo J, et al. Echocardiographic evidence of the cardiac stress of competing in ultra-endurance exercise. Dtsch Z Sportmed 2014;65(March):93–101.
4. Baggish AL, Yared K, Wang F, et al. The impact of endurance exercise training on left ventricular systolic mechanics. Am J Physiol - Heart Circulatory Physiol 2008;295(3):1109–16.

5. la Gerche A, Heidbüchel H, Burns AT, et al. Disproportionate exercise load and remodeling of the athlete's right ventricle. Med Sci Sports Exerc 2011; 43(6):974–81.

6. D'Ascenzi F, Pisicchio C, Caselli S, et al. RV remodeling in Olympic athletes. JACC: Cardiovasc Imaging 2017. https://doi.org/10.1016/j.jcmg.2016.03.017.

7. Zaidi A, Sharma S. Arrhythmogenic right ventricular remodelling in endurance athletes: Pandora's box or Achilles' heel? Eur Heart J 2015;36(30):1955–7.

8. La Gerche A, Burns AT, Mooney DJ, et al. Exercise-induced right ventricular dysfunction and structural remodelling in endurance athletes. Eur Heart J 2012;33(8):998–1006.

9. la Gerche A, Robberecht C, Kuiperi C, et al. Lower than expected desmosomal gene mutation prevalence in endurance athletes with complex ventricular arrhythmias of right ventricular origin. Heart 2010; 96(16):1268–74.

10. Page MJ, McKenzie JE, Bossuyt PM, et al. The PRISMA 2020 statement: an updated guideline for reporting systematic reviews. BMJ 2021;372. https://doi.org/10.1136/bmj.n71.

11. Elliott AD, Gerche A la. The right ventricle following prolonged endurance exercise: are we overlooking the more important side of the heart? A meta-analysis. doi:10.1136/bjsports-2014-093895

12. Huedo-Medina TB, Sánchez-Meca J, Marín-Martínez F, et al. Assessing heterogeneity in meta-analysis: Q statistic or I2 Index? Psychol Methods 2006;11(2):193–206.

13. Egger M, Smith GD, Schneider M, et al. Bias in meta-analysis detected by a simple, graphical test. Br Med J 1997;315(7109):629–34.

14. Dávila-Román VG, Guest TM, Tuteur PG, et al. Transient right but not left ventricular dysfunction after strenuous exercise at high altitude. J Am Coll Cardiol 1997;30(2):468–73.

15. la Gerche A, Rakhit DJ, Claessen G. Exercise and the right ventricle: a potential Achilles' heel. Cardiovasc Res 2017;113(12):1499–508.

16. D'Andrea A, Riegler L, Golia E, et al. Range of right heart measurements in top-level athletes: the training impact. Int J Cardiol 2013;164(1):48–57.

17. Buchan TA, Wright SP, Esfandiari S, et al. Pulmonary hemodynamic and right ventricular responses to brief and prolonged exercise in middle-aged endurance athletes. Am J Physiol - Heart Circulatory Physiol 2019;316(2):H326–34.

18. Lord R, George K, Somauroo J, et al. Alterations in cardiac mechanics following ultra-endurance exercise: insights from left and right ventricular area-deformation loops. J Am Soc Echocardiogr 2016;29(9):879–87.e1.

19. Sanz De La Garza M, Grazioli G, Bijnens BH, et al. Inter-individual variability in right ventricle adaptation after an endurance race. Eur J Prev Cardiol 2016;23(10):1114–24.

20. Mousavi N, Czarnecki A, Kumar K, et al. Relation of biomarkers and cardiac magnetic resonance imaging after marathon running. Am J Cardiol 2009; 103(10):1467–72.

21. Zaidi A, Sheikh N, Jongman JK, et al. Clinical differentiation between physiological remodeling and arrhythmogenic right ventricular cardiomyopathy in athletes with marked electrocardiographic repolarization anomalies. J Am Coll Cardiol 2015;65(25): 2702–11.

22. Douglas PS, O'Toole ML, Miller WDB, et al. Different effects of prolonged exercise on the right and left ventricles. J Am Coll Cardiol 1990;15(1):64–9.

23. Carrio I, Serra-Grima R, Martinez-Duncker C, et al. Transient alterations in cardiac performance following a six hour race. Am J Cardiol 1990; 65(22):1471–4.

24. Neilan TG, Yoerger DM, Douglas PS, et al. Persistent and reversible cardiac dysfunction among amateur marathon runners. Eur Heart J 2006; 27(9):1079–84.

25. Neilan TG, Januzzi JL, Lee-Lewandrowski E, et al. Myocardial injury and ventricular dysfunction related to training levels among nonelite participants in the Boston Marathon. Circulation 2006;114(22): 2325–33.

26. Neilan TG, Ton-Nu TT, Jassal DS, et al. Myocardial adaptation to short-term high-intensity exercise in highly trained athletes. J Am Soc Echocardiogr 2006;19(10):1280–5.

27. Oxborough D, Shave R, Middleton N, et al. The impact of marathon running upon ventricular function as assessed by 2D, Doppler, and tissue-Doppler echocardiography. Echocardiography 2006;23(8):635–41.

28. La Gerche A, Connelly KA, Mooney DJ, et al. Biochemical and functional abnormalities of left and right ventricular function after ultra-endurance exercise. Heart 2008;94(7):860–6.

29. Trivax JE, Franklin BA, Goldstein JA, et al. Acute cardiac effects of marathon running. J Appl Physiol 2010;108(5):1148–53.

30. O'Hanlon R, Wilson M, Wage R, et al. Troponin release following endurance exercise: is inflammation the cause? A cardiovascular magnetic resonance study. J Cardiovasc Magn Reson 2010; 12(1):1–7.

31. Oxborough D, Shave R, Warburton D, et al. Dilatation and dysfunction of the right ventricle immediately after ultraendurance exercise: exploratory insights from conventional two-dimensional and speckle tracking echocardiography. Circ Cardiovasc Imaging 2011;4(3):253–63.

32. Oomah SR, Mousavi N, Bhullar N, et al. The role of three-dimensional echocardiography in the assessment of right ventricular dysfunction after a half marathon: comparison with cardiac magnetic

resonance imaging. J Am Soc Echocardiogr 2011; 24(2):207–13.

33. Karlstedt E, Chelvanathan A, da Silva M, et al. The impact of repeated marathon running on cardiovascular function in the aging population. J Cardiovasc Magn Reson 2012;14(1):1–7.

34. Schattke S, Wagner M, Hättasch R, et al. Single beat 3D echocardiography for the assessment of right ventricular dimension and function after endurance exercise: intraindividual comparison with magnetic resonance imaging. Cardiovasc Ultrasound 2012; 10(1):1–9.

35. Claessen G, Claus P, Ghysels S, et al. Right ventricular fatigue developing during endurance exercise: an exercise cardiac magnetic resonance study. Med Sci Sports Exerc 2014;46(9):1717–26.

36. Lord R, Somauroo J, Stembridge M, et al. The right ventricle following ultra-endurance exercise: insights from novel echocardiography and 12-lead electrocardiography. Eur J Appl Physiol 2015;115(1): 71–80.

37. Maufrais C, Millet GP, Schuster I, et al. Progressive and biphasic cardiac responses during extreme mountain ultramarathon. Am J Physiol - Heart Circulatory Physiol 2016;310(10):H1340–8.

38. Stewart GM, Chan J, Yamada A, et al. Impact of high-intensity endurance exercise on regional left and right ventricular myocardial mechanics. Eur Heart J Cardiovasc Imaging 2017;18(6):688–96.

39. Gajda R, Kowalik E, Rybka S, et al. Evaluation of the heart function of swimmers subjected to exhaustive repetitive endurance efforts during a 500-km relay. Front Physiol 2019;10(MAR):1–9.

40. Martinez V, la Garza MS de, Grazioli G, et al. Cardiac performance after an endurance open water swimming race. Eur J Appl Physiol 2019;119(4):961–70.

41. Christou GA, Pagourelias ED, Anifanti MA, et al. Exploring the determinants of the cardiac changes after ultra-long duration exercise: the echocardiographic Spartathlon study. Eur J Prev Cardiol 2020;27(14):1467–77.

42. Coates AM, King TJ, Currie KD, et al. Alterations in cardiac function following endurance exercise are not duration dependent. Front Physiol 2020; 11(September). https://doi.org/10.3389/fphys.2020. 581797.

43. Chen H, Warncke ML, Muellerleile K, et al. Acute impact of an endurance race on biventricular and biatrial myocardial strain in competitive male and female triathletes evaluated by feature-tracking CMR. Eur Radiol 2021. https://doi.org/10.1007/s00330-021-08401-y. 0123456789.

The International Criteria for Electrocardiogram Interpretation in Athletes
Common Pitfalls and Future Directions

Bradley J. Petek, MD[a,b], Jonathan A. Drezner, MD[c],
Timothy W. Churchill, MD[a,b],*

KEYWORDS

- Athlete • Preparticipation screening • Cardiac screening • Electrocardiography
- Sudden cardiac death

KEY POINTS

- The International Criteria for electrocardiogram (ECG) interpretation is the current standard of care for preparticipation ECG screening in young competitive athletes.
- Common pitfalls using the International Criteria include incorrect interpretation of inferior T-wave inversions, black athlete repolarization patterns, pathologic Q waves, and borderline ECG criteria.
- Future directions to consider for new ECG screening criteria include expanding age/sex/geographic origin-specific ECG changes, addressing low QRS voltage criteria and QRS fragmentation, defining nuanced preventricular contraction (PVC) and ST-segment depression morphology, and providing interpretation guidance when beat-to-beat variation is present.

INTRODUCTION

Preparticipation cardiovascular screening (PPCS) in young competitive athletes is performed to detect conditions associated with sudden cardiac death (SCD). Many medical societies and sports governing bodies recommend PPCS consisting of a focused history and physical examination (H&P) and 12-lead electrocardiogram (ECG).[1–6] Initial ECG screening was criticized for high false-positive rates that led to substantial costs associated with secondary testing and unnecessary (temporary) restriction of athletes from participation. This led to substantial efforts by the scientific community to better understand the difference between physiologic and pathologic ECG findings in athletes. Beginning with the 2010 European Society of Cardiology (ESC) guidelines, several iterations of ECG interpretation standards have emerged, culminating in the most updated ECG interpretation criteria, the International Criteria.[7–12] Since the initial publication of the International Criteria in 2017, multiple studies have shown improved diagnostic accuracy (improved specificity without compromising sensitivity) in different athletic populations. In this review, we present common pitfalls for ECG interpretation in athletes using the International Criteria and highlight future directions to consider in subsequent iterations of ECG screening standards.

EVOLUTION OF ELECTROCARDIOGRAM SCREENING CRITERIA IN ATHLETES

ECG screening among athletic populations first emerged with a New England Journal of Medicine

[a] Division of Cardiology, Massachusetts General Hospital, 55 Fruit Street, Boston, MA 02114, USA;
[b] Cardiovascular Performance Program, Massachusetts General Hospital, Yawkey Suite 5B, 55 Fruit Street, Boston, MA 02114, USA; [c] University of Washington Medical Center for Sports Cardiology, Massachusetts General Hospital, 3800 Montlake Boulevard Northeast, Box 354060, Seattle, WA 98195, USA
* Corresponding author. Cardiovascular Performance Program, Massachusetts General Hospital, Yawkey Suite 5B, 55 Fruit Street, Boston, MA 02114.
E-mail address: twchurchill@partners.org
Twitter: @TimChurchillMD (T.W.C.)

Cardiol Clin 41 (2023) 35–49
https://doi.org/10.1016/j.ccl.2022.08.003
0733-8651/23/© 2022 Elsevier Inc. All rights reserved.

publication by Corrado and colleagues on ECG screening for hypertrophic cardiomyopathy in young athletes.[13] This was followed several years later by a broader and more systematic approach proposed by the ESC in 2005[10] with the publication of the first standardized ECG screening criteria in athletes, and multiple subsequent iterations have followed.[7–12] The initial ESC 2005 criteria provided a list of "abnormal" ECG findings in athletes that warranted further evaluation. A series of National Collegiate Athletic Association articles using these criteria found high rates of abnormal ECGs and false-positive rates (>10%),[14–17] which led to increased scrutiny of how ECG screening may lead to unnecessary secondary testing and significant costs on the medical system. The ESC subsequently proposed new criteria in 2010 that introduced the concept of "common/training-related" ECG patterns, in contrast to more concerning "uncommon/training-unrelated" findings.[7] Although the incorporation of normal training-related ECG findings improved the diagnostic performance of ECG interpretation in athletes, studies using these criteria reported high rates of abnormal ECGs (3%–47%) and false-positive rates (5%–60%) depending on the patient population assessed.[9,18–34] One of the notable features of these criteria was that they were derived from largely Caucasian cohorts and accordingly did not account for emerging data describing common repolarization abnormalities among Black athletes.[35]

The Seattle Criteria were created in 2013 to update interpretation standards inclusive of ethnic-specific ECG findings and provide a pragmatic approach for the sports medicine and cardiology communities.[8] A major addition in this iteration was the recognition that convex (domed) ST elevations followed by T wave inversion (TWI) in V1 to V4 represents a normal, nonpathologic finding in Black athletes.[35] The Seattle criteria also presented important changes in definitions of pathologic Q waves, TWI, ST-segment depressions, left axis deviation, right axis deviation, ventricular preexcitation, short QT, Brugada syndrome, nonspecific intraventricular conduction delay, and arrhythmias. These criteria significantly improved false-positive rates, reported between 2% and 22% depending on the population studied.[9,19,25,26,30,32,36,37]

After the publication of the Seattle Criteria, subsequent studies showed that isolated voltage criteria for atrial enlargement and axis deviation correlated poorly with underlying cardiac disorders in asymptomatic athletes.[38] This recognition led to publication of the Refined Criteria in 2014, which included a borderline group of ECG patterns

(left atrial enlargement, right atrial enlargement, left axis deviation, right axis deviation, right ventricular hypertrophy, Black athlete repolarization pattern), whereby the presence of 2 or more borderline ECG findings warranted further evaluation.[9] With this change, the Refined Criteria once again lowered the reported false-positive rate to 3% to 16%.[9,25,30,39]

The International Criteria are the most recent iteration of ECG interpretation guidelines in athletes and were created in 2017 by an international panel of experts in cardiology and sports medicine.[11] Notable changes in the International Criteria included a change in the definition for pathologic Q waves, recognition of juvenile TWI in V1 to V3 as a normal finding in athletes aged younger than 16 years, and addition of epsilon waves and TWI 1 mm or greater in V5 or V6 alone to the "abnormal" category.[40] Multiple large-scale screening studies have assessed the diagnostic accuracy of the International Criteria and have reported lower false-positive rates ranging from 1.3% to 6.8%.[25,26,41–43] Notably, one of the higher reported false-positive rates (6.8%) was reported in a 2019 study, by McClean and colleagues, which included 1304 Arab and Black athletes in Qatar, highlighting the need for ongoing study to better refine ECG criteria across diverse populations.[26] In contrast, Hyde and colleagues reported a false-positive rate of only 1.3% among 5258 college athletes with application of the International Criteria by sports cardiology experts.[41] Several subsequent studies have been performed in unique demographic populations and sporting disciplines to further characterize the utility of the International Criteria in specific athlete cohorts and have identified populations where the ECG criteria perform well and others that may require further refinement.[22,25,26,41–73]

COMMON PITFALLS

Although the publication of the International Criteria has significantly reduced false-positive rates for ECG interpretation in athletes, there are still ECG patterns that are frequently misclassified by clinicians, particularly those without experience in the interpretation of athlete ECGs. Multiple previous studies have shown that physicians with limited experience in ECG interpretation in athletes will incorrectly classify a large proportion of normal ECGs in athletes as abnormal,[74–77] which can lead to downstream costs from secondary testing and unnecessary sport restriction and psychosocial burden on athletes.[77] However, when physicians are instructed to use a standardized ECG interpretation tool, there is improved accuracy.[60,75]

Table 1
Common pitfalls of electrocardiogram interpretation in athletes using the International Criteria

ECG Abnormality	Common Pitfalls
Inferior TWI	Classified as abnormal with TWI in lead III plus aVF or lead II. Per the International Criteria, TWI in lead III is not considered abnormal; thus, abnormal inferior TWI requires TWI in both lead II and aVF (**Fig. 1**)
Black athlete repolarization pattern	ECGs are classified as abnormal, which have a physiologic Black athlete repolarization pattern consisting of J-point elevation with convex ST-segment elevation and TWI confined to V1–V4 (**Fig. 2**). Extension of TWI into V5 is an abnormal finding and not part of the Black athlete repolarization pattern
Pathologic Q waves	Classified as abnormal when the Q wave is long and thin but does not meet newer criteria including a Q/R > 0.25 or Q wave >40 ms duration (**Fig. 3**)
Borderline ECG findings	Athletes with 1 borderline ECG finding (eg, axis deviation, atrial enlargement, or complete RBBB) are flagged as abnormal when the International Criteria requires 2 borderline findings (**Fig. 4**)

In studies which have compared local ECG interpretation to an expert overread, ECG findings that are commonly misinterpreted by local providers as abnormal include: LVH (left ventricular hypertrophy), nonpathologic TWI, isolated axis deviation, IVCD less than 140 milliseconds, RBBB in isolation, misinterpreted accessory pathway, nonpathologic rhythm variants, PVCs (<2 per strip), first-degree AV block, and J-waves.[45,47] In contrast, ECG findings classified as normal by local providers but readjudicated as abnormal by expert overread include: pathologic TWI, biatrial enlargement, pathologic Q waves, pathologic ST-segment depressions, and atrial tachyarrhythmias.[45,47] These studies highlight the importance of continual medical education for clinicians using ECG in the cardiovascular care of athletes. This education can occur via in-person educational courses with content experts, online training courses (https://uwsportscardiology.org/e-academy/), or other educational materials. An overview of commonly misclassified ECG abnormalities using the International Criteria for ECG interpretation is presented in **Table 1**. Examples of ECGs commonly misclassified are presented in **Figs. 1–4**.

FUTURE DIRECTIONS

Although the International Criteria outperform all previous ECG interpretation standards in athletes, there is scope for improvement as new evidence emerges (**Table 2**). Ideally, ECG interpretation criteria would be individualized for the demographic and sport of each athlete. However, making the criteria too complex also limits the ease of use and application in everyday practice. Therefore, trade-offs are needed that maximize sensitivity/specificity in unique populations but also maintain user-friendly criteria, particularly when applied outside of expert centers. In the following sections, we present future considerations for subsequent ECG interpretation standards.

Race/Ethnicity/Geographic Origin-Specific Electrocardiogram Criteria

The first race-specific ECG criterion was the Black athlete repolarization pattern (convex/"domed" ST elevations followed by TWI in V1–V4) included in the 2013 Seattle Criteria, given the absence of pathologic findings in studies performing comprehensive cardiovascular testing in athletes with this pattern.[11,35] Although the recognition of this pattern reduced false-positive rates, the use of race to delineate all Black athletes has recently been challenged. In a study by Riding and colleagues involving 1698 mixed sport athletes, the authors observed significant differences in benign TWI patterns (V1–V4) in Black athletes based on geographic origin (Middle African 11.8%, West African 5.3%, African-American/Caribbean 2.4%, East African 1.5%, North African 0%).[72] The authors conclude that because there is heterogeneity in the prevalence of benign TWI patterns between the athlete cohorts, larger subgroups based on

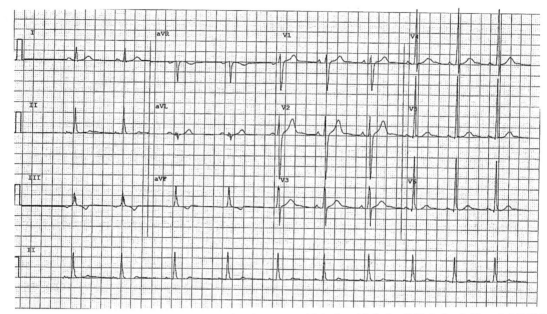

Fig. 1. Common Pitfalls—Inferior TWIs. Example of an ECG with isolated inferior TWIs in leads III and aVF. This ECG is considered normal per the International criteria. Given TWI in III is considered normal, inferior TWI need to be present in both II and aVF to be considered abnormal.

geographic origin should be studied before it is concluded that this repolarization pattern can be generalized to all Black athletes.

This repolarization pattern has also been characterized in non-Black athletes. Calore and colleagues compared anterior TWI in 80 athletes (66% Black) to 153 patients with hypertrophic or arrhythmogenic cardiomyopathy.[78] Cardiomyopathy was completely excluded in athletes with a combination of J-point elevation 1 mm or greater and TWI not extending beyond V4, regardless of race. These findings require additional investigation in larger cohorts of athletes with different race/ethnicity and geographic origin.

Since the publication of the International Criteria in 2017, multiple subsequent studies assessed these criteria in populations of athletes from all over the world including the United

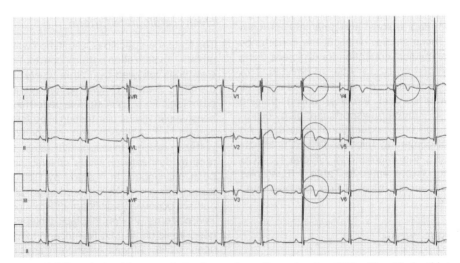

Fig. 2. Common Pitfalls—Black athlete repolarization pattern. Example of an ECG with a Black athlete repolarization pattern (J point elevation with convex ST elevation and TWIs confined to V1–V4—denoted here with *blue circles*). This ECG is considered normal per the International Criteria. TWIs extending into V5 are always considered abnormal.

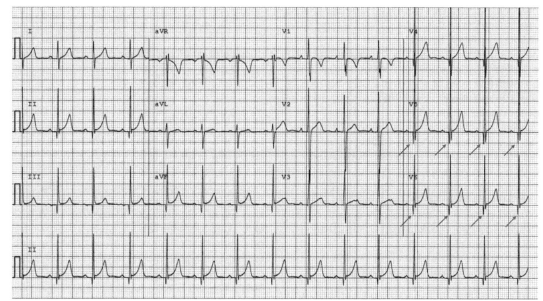

Fig. 3. Common Pitfalls—Nonpathologic Q waves. Example of an ECG with Q waves greater than 3 mm in the lateral leads (*blue arrows*). This ECG is normal per the International Criteria, given the International Criteria requires Q/R ratio of 0.25 or greater or q of 40 milliseconds or greater in 2 or more leads (excluding III and aVR).

States,[41,42,44–49] the United Kingdom,[22,25,50–52] the Netherlands,[53] Macedonia,[54] Poland,[55] Italy,[43,56–58] Switzerland,[43,59,60] China,[61] Malaysia,[62–64] Pacific Islands,[65,66] Ecuador,[67] Argentina,[68] Qatar,[26,72,79] Ghana,[69,73] Cameroon,[70] and Nigeria.[71] Within these, rates of abnormal ECGs based on the International Criteria have varied widely. Athlete cohorts with high rates of abnormal ECGs have included Ghanian male soccer players (23.3%),[73] Malaysian male soccer players (20%),[64] United States National Basketball Association male players (15.6%),[46] Cameroonian

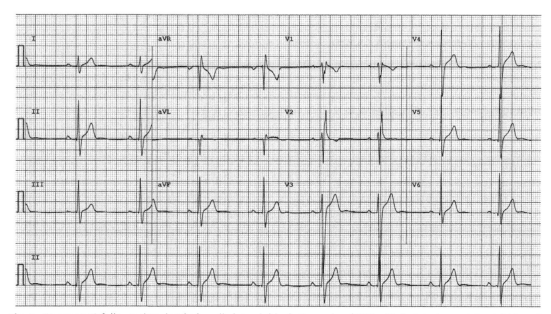

Fig. 4. Common Pitfalls—Isolated right bundle branch block. Example of ECG with isolated complete right bundle branch block. QRS axis does not meet International Criteria threshold for right axis deviation ($\geq$120°). This ECG would be considered as normal per the International Criteria given that only one borderline criteria is present and there are no other abnormal findings.

male ultramarathoners (13.6%),[70] Middle African male athletes from the Qatar Olympic Committee (11.9%),[72] United States national team female soccer players (11.5%),[44] and Caucasian male professional cyclists (9.3%).[59] In contrast, populations with low rates of abnormal ECGs include US collegiate athletes (1.5%–2.1%)[41,42,45,48] and UK soccer players (1.8%).[25]

Given this persistent heterogeneity, it is clear that the generation of high-quality data from a diverse collection of source populations is required, with an emphasis on data defining not only race but geographic origin when possible. Such data will allow future iterations of ECG interpretation criteria to more explicitly consider race/ethnicity and geographic origins in the creation of specific recommendations.

Age-Specific Electrocardiogram Criteria

Previous iterations of ECG screening criteria have been developed for the screening of asymptomatic athletes aged older than 12 years and younger than 35 years.[8,11] More research is needed to understand if the International Criteria can be applied to younger athletes aged less than 12 years or if specific modifications of the criteria are needed. Preliminary studies have shown that these ECG screening criteria may also be effective in Master's athletes (age >35 years).[53] As the International Criteria have been specifically curated for athletes aged 35 years or younger, extrapolation to older populations requires additional study and consideration.

Sex-Specific Electrocardiogram Criteria

Although it is well established that female athletes have different ECG features compared with male athletes,[80] the only sex-specific recommendation in the International Criteria pertains to cutpoints for an abnormal corrected QT segment (QTc), defined in female athletes as 480 milliseconds or greater and in male athletes as 470 milliseconds or greater. Of specific interest in the screening setting is that female athletes, especially female endurance athletes, frequently have a higher percentage of anterior TWI (V1–V3). In studies assessing sex-based differences in ECG patterns, the prevalence of anterior TWI in female athletes ranges from 2% to 9%,[25,44,81–83] and anterior TWI in this population are unlikely to represent underlying cardiac pathologic condition.[25,44,83] Therefore, the presence of anterior TWI in female athletes may be a normal finding not warranting additional investigation. It has also been speculated that ECG lead placement may differ between male and female athletes due to the presence of breast tissue, particularly in the setting of large screening events in which ECGs are often not performed in completely private environments. Added consideration of sex differences in the interpretation of anterior TWI thus represents an important focus for future research.

Low QRS Voltage

Low QRS voltage is typically defined as a QRS amplitude of less than 0.5 mV in all 6 limb leads or less than 1 mV in the precordial leads.[84] Other definitions including the total sum of limb leads less than 3.0 mV have also been used. However, low voltage should also be considered in those with significant interval decreases in QRS voltage on 2 consecutive ECGs, in which case, the difference may suggest interval development of a pathologic condition. Although low voltage can be secondary to many cardiac and noncardiac causes (eg, obesity, emphysema), in competitive athletes important causes of SCD, which may demonstrate low QRS voltage, include arrhythmogenic right ventricular cardiomyopathy (ARVC),[85] myocarditis,[86] nonischemic LV scar, and infiltrative cardiac diseases. These conditions have increased electrical impedance where replacement fibrosis and the loss of electrically active myocardial mass lead to low QRS voltages.

Recent studies have suggested that a low voltage QRS can help differentiate ARVC from electrocardiographic remodeling in athletes.[87,88] In a study by Brosnan and colleagues of 100 healthy athletes matched with 100 ARVC patients both with TWI in at least 2 anterior ECG leads (V1-V4), the ARVC patients had a greater prevalence of low voltage in the limb leads (21% vs 1%, $P < .001$), as well as more frequent precordial TWI beyond V3 (34% vs 8%, $P < .001$), inferior TWI (31% vs 3%, $P < .001$), and PVCs (18% vs 0%, $P < .001$).[88] The authors conclude that low QRS voltages may be an additional finding to differentiate healthy athletes from those with ARVC. A subsequent study by Finocchiaro and colleagues replicated this finding, comparing 162 patients with ARVC to 129 young controls with anterior TWI, again demonstrating an increased prevalence of low limb lead QRS voltage in the ARVC patients compared with controls (15% vs 4%, $P = .01$).[87] Among Olympic athletes (n = 516), Mango and colleagues found low QRS amplitude, defined here as either QRS amplitude of less than 0.5 mV in all 6 limb leads or less than 1 mV in the precordial leads, to be present in 4% of athletes but did not find any significant associations with pathologic condition.[89] In another recent study, Zorzi and colleagues compared the prevalence

Table 2
Future directions of electrocardiogram interpretation in athletes

ECG Parameters	Future Considerations
Age/sex/geographic origin	Optimization of ECG criteria in diverse populations
PVC morphology	Consideration of the frequency of PVCs in conjunction with PVC morphology as "benign" or "malignant" (eg, 1 malignant PVC vs multiple benign PVCs warrants additional investigation)
Low QRS voltage	Consideration of adding low QRS voltage criteria given association with ARVC, myocarditis, nonischemic LV scar, and infiltrative myocardial diseases
QRS fragmentation	Consideration of QRS fragmentation as a potential borderline finding because this parameter has been associated with multiple pathologic cardiovascular conditions in the general population
ST-segment depression morphology	Consideration of ST-segment depression morphology (eg, horizontal or downsloping [but not upsloping] warrants additional investigation)

(continued on next page)

Table 2
(continued)

ECG Parameters	Future Considerations
Borderline ECG findings	Further understanding on which combination of findings predict underlying pathologic condition
Beat-to-beat variation	Guidance on how to interpret abnormal ECG findings if only present in a subset of beats in any specific lead (eg, abnormal if >50% of beats)

of low QRS voltage in the limb leads (all <0.5 mV) between Italian athletes (n = 2229), Black athletes (n = 1115), general population patients (n = 1115), and patients with known arrhythmogenic cardiomyopathy (AC) or nonischemic LV scar (NILVS, n = 58).[90] The key finding of this article was a low prevalence of low QRS voltage in athletes compared with the AC and NILVS patients (1.1% vs 12%). In addition, the authors also noted that 2/5 (40%) athletes with low QRS and exercise-induced ventricular arrhythmias were found to have a cardiomyopathy on cardiac MRI (1 AC, 1 NILVS). The authors therefore conclude that low QRS voltage should be considered in future iterations of ECG screening criteria.

Low QRS voltage has also been found in patients with myocarditis in the general population.[91] Additional study is required to define the clinical implications of low QRS voltage and to determine whether it merits inclusion in future iterations of ECG interpretation criteria.

QRS Fragmentation

Fragmentation of a narrow QRS is defined as the presence of an additional R wave (R'), notching in the nadir of the S wave or the presence of greater than 1 R' in 2 contiguous leads (**Fig. 5**).[92] Conversely, fragmentation of a wide complex QRS has been defined as greater than 2 R waves (R''), more than 2 notches in the R wave, or more than 2 notches in the downstroke or upstroke of the S wave.[92] Previous studies have shown that QRS fragmentation is associated with and often predicts poor prognosis in many cardiac diseases

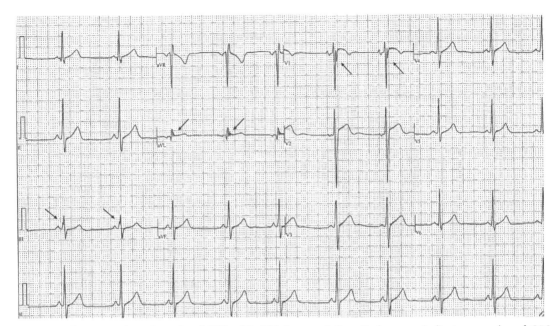

Fig. 5. QRS fragmentation. Example of ECG with QRS fragmentation. Red arrows indicate examples of QRS fragmentation.

including chronic coronary artery disease (myocardial scar),[93] dilated cardiomyopathy,[94] ARVC,[95] cardiac sarcoidosis,[96] and Brugada syndrome.[97] Of specific interest in the athletic populations would be if flagging QRS fragmentation aids in the detection of cardiomyopathies during PPCS.

Although QRS fragmentation has been associated with ARVC, the diagnostic performance of this finding seems to be limited. Notably, this ECG abnormality has not been included in the current or previous diagnostic criteria for ARVC.[98,99]

Limited studies have assessed the utility of QRS fragmentation in the diagnosis of underlying cardiac disorders in athletes. Recent study by Ollitrault and colleagues demonstrated that QRS fragmentation in V1 (fQRS$_{V1}$) was more common in athletes than nonathletes (22% vs 5%, $P < .001$). Within this group, athletes with fQRS$_{V1}$ (n = 26) showed significant structural differences compared with athletes without fQRS$_{V1}$ (n = 93), including greater indexed right ventricular outflow tract (RVOT) dimensions, indexed RV basal diameter, tricuspid annular planar systolic excursion, indexed LV end diastolic diameter, and indexed LV mass.[100] The authors therefore conclude that fQRS$_{V1}$ is common among healthy athletes and may be considered a sign of RV remodeling, although this study did not provide any broader clinical or genetic correlation. Although this study suggests QRS fragmentation is common in healthy athletes and may not be a good distinguisher of disease, this study focused on QRS fragmentation in lead V1 only and larger scale studies are needed

because earlier studies comparing ECG findings in athletes to patients with ARVC have not reported the presence or absence of QRS fragmentation.[87,88] Although QRS fragmentation is easily recognizable, it remains unknown if it would provide additive diagnostic value above and beyond the current criteria.

Premature Ventricular Contractions

The current International Criteria recommend further evaluation for all athletes who have 2 or greater premature ventricular contractions (PVCs) on a 10-second ECG.[11] Although PVCs can be a marker of myocardial disease, the chosen cutoff is arbitrary and does not consider PVC morphology, which can be an important diagnostic and prognostic marker.[101]

The morphology of PVCs can help to identify the anatomic origin of the ectopic beats, which has important implications for the likelihood of underlying cardiovascular disease. In athletes, infundibular right ventricular outflow tract and left ventricular outflow tract (RVOT and LVOT) and fascicular (left anterior and posterior) PVC origins are frequently seen and usually considered to be benign. RVOT PVCs are characterized by an LBBB pattern, inferior axis, and late precordial transition (R/s = 1 after V3; **Fig. 6**), whereas LVOT PVCs are characterized by an LBBB pattern, inferior axis, and early precordial transition (R/s = 1 by V2 or V3). Fascicular PVCs are characterized by a typical RBBB and QRS duration less than

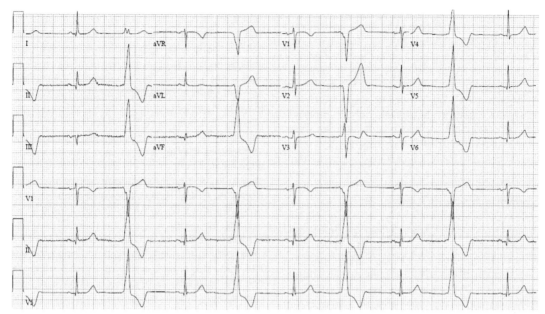

Fig. 6. RVOT PVCs. Example of ECG with RVOT PVCs. Pertinent features include left bundle branch block pattern, inferior axis, and late precordial transition. RVOTs are broadly considered more likely to have a benign course.

130 milliseconds (anterior = inferior axis, posterior = superior axis). In contrast, patterns concerning for underlying myocardial disease in athletes include an atypical RBBB with QRS 130 milliseconds or greater (suggestive of mitral valve annulus, papillary muscles, or left ventricular sites of origin; **Fig. 7**) or an LBBB pattern with superior or intermediate axis (right ventricular free wall, interventricular septum).[102]

The prevalence of PVCs in young competitive athletes versus sedentary controls has been evaluated in many studies with mixed results.[103–107]

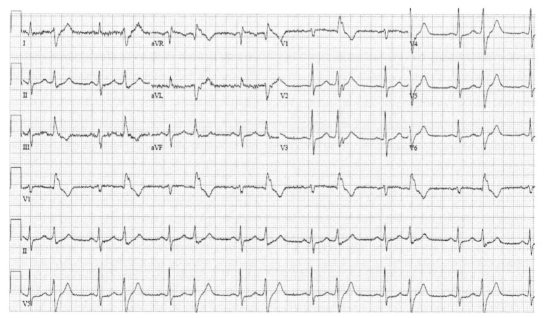

Fig. 7. Papillary muscle PVCs. Example of ECG with PVCs originating from papillary muscle. Note the atypical right bundle branch block pattern with wide (≥130 milliseconds) QRS. This PVC morphology is more often associated with myocardial disease and increased risk for malignant clinical course.

Most studies were in small populations and have shown similar overall burden of PVCs in athletes as in control populations.[103,104,106] However, in a recent study by Zorzi and colleagues assessing the burden of PVCs and arrhythmias in athletes (n = 288) versus controls (n = 144), the presence of 1 or greater PVC on 24-hour 12-lead ECG monitoring was higher in the athlete cohort (59% vs 40%, P < .0001).[107] Although athletes may have a higher prevalence of PVCs depending on the study, studies have consistently shown that frequent or complex ventricular arrhythmias (couplets, triplets, or NSVT) seem rare in young competitive athletes (6%–13%).[103–108]

Given these collective findings, a limitation in the current International Criteria is that recommendations for additional testing are based on the quantity of PVCs on a 12-lead ECG without consideration of the PVC morphology. An athlete could have 1 PVC from a concerning origin (eg, LBBB with superior or intermediate axis) and not undergo further evaluation for structural heart disease, whereas another athlete with 2 PVCs of outflow tract or fascicular origin may undergo an extensive workup when underlying disease is unlikely. Future iterations of ECG screening criteria should consider the addition of PVC morphology in some form, and research should assess the combined diagnostic effect of PVC morphology and PVC burden on the surface ECG in the PPCS setting.

ST-Segment Depressions

Current International Criteria recommendations consider an ECG abnormal if there are ST-segment depressions 0.5 mm or greater in 2 or more contiguous leads.[11] ST-depressions are frequently a marker of underlying myocardial disease and can be found in conditions leading to SCD in young competitive athletes such as hypertrophic cardiomyopathy.[109,110] However, the current guidelines do not specifically comment on ST-segment depression morphology (eg, upsloping, horizontal, or downsloping) as a component of this assessment, likely because prior studies in athletes have focused on the presence or absence of ST-segment depressions and have not reported the morphology of the ST changes in detail. Given that ST-segment depressions are generally considered abnormal and possibly associated with pathologic condition in the general population when they are horizontal or downsloping, research is needed to determine if upsloping ST-segment depressions among athletes truly warrants more evaluation or if it could be considered a normal or borderline finding.

Borderline Findings

The International Criteria currently includes a section of "borderline" ECG abnormalities (left atrial enlargement, right atrial enlargement, left axis deviation, right axis deviation, complete RBBB) where 2 or more abnormalities in this category are needed to warrant further testing.[11] The borderline category was created to account for the findings of the seminal study by Gati and colleagues, which demonstrated that athletes with isolated axis deviation or atrial enlargement (n = 579) did not have any major structural or functional abnormalities on TTE.[38] Complete RBBB patterns are also included in the borderline category on the basis of a study of 510 US athletes, which found 2.5% (n = 13) to have a complete RBBB, all of whom were free of pathologic structural heart disease.[111] The authors of this study also subsequently assessed the association of RBBB with pathologic condition from previous athlete studies and found no reported cardiac pathologic condition among asymptomatic athletes with complete RBBB.[112]

Although this group of borderline findings has been a major driver in reducing false-positive interpretations, considerable uncertainty remains regarding whether specific combinations of borderline ECG abnormalities are associated with high-risk conditions or whether certain combinations may actually be considered normal findings. As such, additional research adding granularity to athletes with 2 or more borderline ECG findings would be valuable.

Beat-to-Beat Variation

Although the International Criteria provide a framework for normal and abnormal ECG findings in athletes, a frequently encountered issue not covered in the text is how to handle beat-to-beat variation. When interpreting an athlete's ECG, it is very common that there may be 2 to 3 beats available for each lead that is not included in the rhythm strip. Interpretation of abnormal findings can be difficult if an abnormality is visualized in a subset of the beats available in any specific lead (eg, TWI meets criteria in 1/3 or 2/3 beats). Guidance on how to interpret beat-to-beat variation would be valuable in future iterations of ECG interpretation guidelines. For instance, greater than 50% of the beats in a given lead might be required to define an abnormality as "present." Although published research on this topic is lacking, it seems likely that the proportion of beats with a given finding will have implications for test sensitivity and specificity. For example, if TWI is only required in 1/3 beats to be considered abnormal as opposed to 2/3 or 3/3 beats, this definition may be more sensitive but likely less specific.

SUMMARY

Criteria for the evaluation of the athlete's ECG have evolved considerably during the past 20 years because the scientific understanding of physiologic versus pathologic findings has expanded. With ongoing refinement, metrics of test performance have markedly improved. Nevertheless, important challenges and pitfalls to the application and interpretation of these criteria remain with several important areas of future research identified to fill existing knowledge gaps. Ongoing efforts are required to further refine ECG interpretation standards in athletes.

CLINICS CARE POINTS

- The International Criteria for ECG interpretation in athletes have improved specificity of ECG interpretation in this population. These can be used as a reference at the point of care by clinicians evaluating athlete ECGs.
- Common pitfalls in athlete ECG interpretation that the clinician should be aware of include identification of pathologic inferior T-wave inversions and pathologic Q waves, recognition of the black athlete repolarization pattern, and correct application of the criteria's 'borderline' finding category.
- Normative ECG data specific to the sport and population in question are required, and caution should be exercised applying data from different populations and athletic contexts.
- Other areas requiring additional research include the significance of low QRS voltage and QRS fragmentation, greater granularity regarding the implications of specific PVC morphologies, and more specific guidance regarding beat-to-beat variation in ECG findings.

DISCLOSURE

The authors report no disclosures.

CONFLICT OF INTEREST

The authors report no conflicts of interest.

REFERENCES

1. Ljungqvist A, Jenoure P, Engebretsen L, et al. The international Olympic Committee (IOC) consensus statement on periodic health evaluation of elite athletes March 2009. Br J Sports Med 2009;43(9): 631–43.
2. Mont L, Pelliccia A, Sharma S, et al. Pre-participation cardiovascular evaluation for athletic participants to prevent sudden death: position paper from the EHRA and the EACPR, branches of the ESC. Endorsed by APHRS, HRS, and SOLAECE. Ep Europace 2016;19(1):139–63.
3. Löllgen HBM, Cummiskey J, Bachl N, et al. The pre-participation examination in sports: EFSMA statement on ECG for pre-participation examination. Dtsch Z Sportmed 2015;66:151–5.
4. Dvorak J, Kramer EB, Schmied CM, et al. The FIFA medical emergency bag and FIFA 11 steps to prevent sudden cardiac death: setting a global standard and promoting consistent football field emergency care. Br J Sports Med 2013;47(18): 1199–202.
5. Maron BJ, Levine BD, Washington RL, et al. Eligibility and disqualification recommendations for competitive athletes with cardiovascular abnormalities: task force 2: preparticipation screening for cardiovascular disease in competitive athletes: a scientific statement from the American Heart Association and American College of Cardiology. J Am Coll Cardiol 2015;66(21):2356–61.
6. Drezner JA, O'connor FG, Harmon KG, et al. AMSSM position statement on cardiovascular pre-participation screening in athletes: current evidence, knowledge gaps, recommendations and future directions. Br J Sports Med 2017;51(3): 153–67.
7. Corrado D, Pelliccia A, Heidbuchel H, et al. Recommendations for interpretation of 12-lead electrocardiogram in the athlete. Eur Heart J 2009;31(2): 243–59.
8. Drezner JA, Ackerman MJ, Anderson J, et al. Electrocardiographic interpretation in athletes: the 'Seattle criteria. Br J Sports Med 2013;47(3):122–4.
9. Sheikh N, Papadakis M, Ghani S, et al. Comparison of electrocardiographic criteria for the detection of cardiac abnormalities in elite black and white athletes. Circulation 2014;129(16):1637–49.
10. Corrado D, Pelliccia A, Bjørnstad HH, et al. Cardiovascular pre-participation screening of young competitive athletes for prevention of sudden death: proposal for a common European protocol: consensus statement of the study group of sport cardiology of the working group of cardiac Rehabilitation and exercise Physiology and the working group of myocardial and Pericardial diseases of the European society of cardiology. Eur Heart J 2005;26(5):516–24.
11. Drezner JA, Sharma S, Baggish A, et al. International criteria for electrocardiographic interpretation in athletes: consensus statement. Br J Sports Med 2017;51(9):704–31.

12. Corrado D, Biffi A, Basso C, et al. 12-lead ECG in the athlete: physiological versus pathological abnormalities. Br J Sports Med 2009;43(9):669–76.

13. Corrado D, Basso C, Schiavon M, et al. Screening for hypertrophic cardiomyopathy in young athletes. New Engl J Med 1998;339(6):364–9.

14. Baggish AL, Hutter AM, Wang F, et al. Cardiovascular screening in college athletes with and without electrocardiography: a cross-sectional study. Ann Intern Med 2010;152(5):269–75.

15. Magalski A, McCoy M, Zabel M, et al. Cardiovascular screening with electrocardiography and echocardiography in collegiate athletes. Am J Med 2011;124(6):511–8.

16. Le V-V, Wheeler MT, Mandic S, et al. Addition of the electrocardiogram to the preparticipation examination of college athletes. Clin J Sport Med 2010; 20(2):98–105.

17. Malhotra R, West JJ, Dent J, et al. Cost and yield of adding electrocardiography to history and physical in screening Division I intercollegiate athletes: a 5-year experience. Heart Rhythm 2011;8(5):721–7.

18. Alattar A, Ghani S, Mahdy N, et al. Pre-participation musculoskeletal and cardiac screening of male athletes in the United Arab Emirates. Transl Med Unisa 2014;9:43.

19. Brosnan M, La Gerche A, Kalman J, et al. The Seattle Criteria increase the specificity of preparticipation ECG screening among elite athletes. Br J Sports Med 2014;48(15):1144–50.

20. Chandra N, Bastiaenen R, Papadakis M, et al. Prevalence of electrocardiographic anomalies in young individuals: relevance to a nationwide cardiac screening program. J Am Coll Cardiol 2014; 63(19):2028–34.

21. Deligiannis AP, Kouidi EJ, Koutlianos NA, et al. Eighteen years' experience applying old and current strategies in the pre-participation cardiovascular screening of athletes. Hellenic J Cardiol 2014; 55(1):32.

22. Dhutia H, Malhotra A, Finocchiaro G, et al. Impact of the international recommendations for electrocardiographic interpretation on cardiovascular screening in young athletes. J Am Coll Cardiol 2017;70(6):805–7.

23. Dunn TP, Pickham D, Aggarwal S, et al. Limitations of current AHA guidelines and proposal of new guidelines for the preparticipation examination of athletes. Clin J Sport Med 2015;25(6):472–7.

24. Fudge J, Harmon KG, Owens DS, et al. Cardiovascular screening in adolescents and young adults: a prospective study comparing the Pre-participation Physical Evaluation Monograph 4th Edition and ECG. Br J Sports Med 2014;48(15):1172–8.

25. Malhotra A, Dhutia H, Yeo T-J, et al. Accuracy of the 2017 international recommendations for clinicians who interpret adolescent athletes' ECGs: a cohort study of 11 168 British white and black soccer players. Br J Sports Med 2019;54(12):739–45.

26. McClean G, Riding NR, Pieles G, et al. Diagnostic accuracy and Bayesian analysis of new international ECG recommendations in paediatric athletes. Heart 2019;105(2):152–9.

27. Menafoglio A, Di Valentino M, Segatto J-M, et al. Costs and yield of a 15-month preparticipation cardiovascular examination with ECG in 1070 young athletes in Switzerland: implications for routine ECG screening. Br J Sports Med 2014;48(15): 1157–61.

28. Pickham D, Zarafshar S, Sani D, et al. Comparison of three ECG criteria for athlete preparticipation screening. J Electrocardiol 2014; 47(6):769–74.

29. Price DE, McWilliams A, Asif IM, et al. Electrocardiography-inclusive screening strategies for detection of cardiovascular abnormalities in high school athletes. Heart Rhythm 2014;11(3):442–9.

30. Riding NR, Sheikh N, Adamuz C, et al. Comparison of three current sets of electrocardiographic interpretation criteria for use in screening athletes. Heart 2015;101(5):384–90.

31. Snoek JA, Jongman JK, Brandon T, et al. Performance of the Lausanne questionnaire and the 2010 European Society of Cardiology criteria for ECG interpretation in athletes. Eur J Prev Cardiol 2015;22(3):397–405.

32. Wasfy MM, DeLuca J, Wang F, et al. ECG findings in competitive rowers: normative data and the prevalence of abnormalities using contemporary screening recommendations. Br J Sports Med 2015;49(3):200–6.

33. Weiner RB, Hutter AM, Wang F, et al. Performance of the 2010 European Society of Cardiology criteria for ECG interpretation in athletes. Heart 2011; 97(19):1573–7.

34. Wilson MG, Chatard J, Carré F, et al. Prevalence of electrocardiographic abnormalities in West-Asian and African male athletes. Br J Sports Med 2012; 46(5):341–7.

35. Papadakis M, Carre F, Kervio G, et al. The prevalence, distribution, and clinical outcomes of electrocardiographic repolarization patterns in male athletes of African/Afro-Caribbean origin. Eur Heart J 2011;32(18):2304–13.

36. Drezner JA, Owens DS, Prutkin JM, et al. Electrocardiographic screening in national collegiate athletic association athletes. Am J Cardiol 2016; 118(5):754–9.

37. Williams EA, Pelto HF, Toresdahl BG, et al. Performance of the American heart association (AHA) 14-point evaluation versus electrocardiography for the cardiovascular screening of high school athletes: a prospective study. J Am Heart Assoc 2019; 8(14):e012235.

38. Gati S, Sheikh N, Ghani S, et al. Should axis deviation or atrial enlargement be categorised as abnormal in young athletes? The athlete's electrocardiogram: time for re-appraisal of markers of pathology. Eur Heart J 2013;34(47):3641–8.
39. Fuller C, Scott C, Hug-English C, et al. Five-year experience with screening electrocardiograms in national collegiate athletic association Division I athletes. Clin J Sport Med 2016;26(5):369.
40. Drezner JA. 18 highlights from the International Criteria for ECG interpretation in athletes. In: BMJ publishing group Ltd and British association of sport and exercise medicine. 2019.
41. Hyde N, Prutkin JM, Drezner JA. Electrocardiogram interpretation in NCAA athletes: comparison of the 'Seattle'and 'International'criteria. J Electrocardiol 2019;56:81–4.
42. Conway JJ, Krystofiak J, Quirolgico K, et al. Evaluation of a prepaticipation cardiovascular screening program among 1,686 national collegiate athletic association Division I athletes: comparison of the Seattle, refined, and international electrocardiogram screening criteria. Clin J Sport Med 2020;32(3):306–12.
43. Halasz G, Cattaneo M, Piepoli M, et al. Pediatric athletes' ECG and diagnostic performance of contemporary ECG interpretation criteria. Int J Cardiol 2021;335:40–6.
44. Churchill TW, Petek BJ, Wasfy MM, et al. Cardiac structure and function in elite female and male soccer players. JAMA Cardiol 2021;6(3):316–25.
45. Petek BJ, Drezner JA, Prutkin JM, et al. Electrocardiogram interpretation in college athletes: local institution versus sports cardiology center interpretation. J Electrocardiol 2020;62:49–56.
46. Waase MP, Mutharasan RK, Whang W, et al. Electrocardiographic findings in national Basketball association athletes. JAMA Cardiol 2018;3(1): 69–74.
47. Weiss M, Rao P, Johnson D, et al. Physician adherence to 'Seattle'and 'International'ECG criteria in adolescent athletes: an analysis of compliance by specialty, experience, and practice environment. J Electrocardiol 2020;60:98–101.
48. Rambarat CA, Reifsteck F, Clugston JR, et al. Preparticipation cardiac evaluation findings in a cohort of collegiate female athletes. Am J Cardiol 2021; 140:134–9.
49. Thomas JA, Perez-Alday E A, Junell A, et al. Vectorcardiogram in athletes: the Sun valley Ski study. Ann Noninvasive Electrocardiol 2019;24(3): e12614.
50. Brown B, Millar L, Somauroo J, et al. Left ventricular remodeling in elite and sub-elite road cyclists. Scand J Med Sci Sports 2020;30(7):1132–9.
51. Malhotra A, Oxborough D, Rao P, et al. Defining the normal Spectrum of electrocardiographic and left ventricular Adaptations in mixed-race male adolescent soccer players. Circulation 2021;143(1):94–6.
52. Morrison B, Mohammad A, Oxborough D, et al. The 12-lead electrocardiogram of the elite female footballer as defined by different interpretation criteria across the competitive season. Eur J Sport Sci 2021;1–24 (just-accepted).
53. Panhuyzen-Goedkoop NM, Wellens HJ, Verbeek AL, et al. ECG criteria for the detection of high-risk cardiovascular conditions in master athletes. Eur J Prev Cardiol 2020;27(14):1529–38.
54. Karagjozova I, Petrovska S, Nikolic S, et al. Frequency of electrocardiographic changes in trained athletes in the Republic of Macedonia. Open access Macedonian J Med Sci 2017;5(6):708.
55. Jakubiak AA, Konopka M, Bursa D, et al. Benefits and limitations of electrocardiographic and echocardiographic screening in top level endurance athletes. Biol Sport 2021;38(1):71.
56. Zorzi A, Calore C, Vio R, et al. Accuracy of the ECG for differential diagnosis between hypertrophic cardiomyopathy and athlete's heart: comparison between the European Society of Cardiology (2010) and International (2017) criteria. Br J Sports Med 2018;52(10):667–73.
57. Calò L, Martino A, Tranchita E, et al. Electrocardiographic and echocardiographic evaluation of a large cohort of peri-pubertal soccer players during pre-participation screening. Eur J Prev Cardiol 2019;26(13):1444–55.
58. Vessella T, Zorzi A, Merlo L, et al. The Italian preparticipation evaluation programme: diagnostic yield, rate of disqualification and cost analysis. Br J Sports Med 2020;54(4):231–7.
59. Beale AL, Julliard MV, Maziarski P, et al. Electrocardiographic findings in elite professional cyclists: the 2017 international recommendations in practice. J Sci Med Sport 2019;22(4):380–4.
60. Schneiter S, Trachsel LD, Perrin T, et al. Interobserver agreement in athletes ECG interpretation using the recent international recommendations for ECG interpretation in athletes among observers with different levels of expertise. PLOS ONE 2018;13(11):e0206072.
61. Wen X, Huang Y-m, Shen T-H, et al. Prevalence of abnormal and borderline electrocardiogram changes in 13, 079 Chinese amateur marathon runners. BMC Sports Sci Med Rehabil 2021; 13(1):1–7.
62. Aziz MA, Hanifah RA. Characteristics OF RESTING ECG among SABAH professional male FOOTBALLERS. Malaysian J Move Health Exerc 2021; 10(1).
63. Lim ZL, Mokhtar AH, Jaffar MR. Pre-participation evaluation of Malaysian university athletes–the importance of cardiovascular screening. Malaysian J Move Health Exerc 2017;6(2).

64. Ariffin F, Khir RN, Mohamed-Yassin M-S, et al. Identifying electrocardiogram pattern changes and Their association with echocardiography among Malaysian Footballers Attending pre-participation evaluation. J Clin Health Sci 2020;5(1):49–59.

65. Chatard J-C, Espinosa F, Donnadieu R, et al. Pre-participation cardiovascular evaluation in Pacific Island athletes. Int J Cardiol 2019;278:273–9.

66. Johnson C, Forsythe L, Somauroo J, et al. Cardiac structure and function in elite native Hawaiian and Pacific Islander Rugby football League athletes: an exploratory study. Int J Cardiovasc Imaging 2018;34(5):725–34.

67. Medrano Plana Y, Castillo Marcillo ÁR, Lugo Morales AM, et al. Alteraciones electrocardiográficas en jóvenes atletas de alto rendimiento. CorSalud 2019;11(4):296–301.

68. Ramognino F, Ferraro F, BLUMBERG ES, et al. Hallazgos electrocardiográficos anormales en deportistas amateur: comparación de los criterios de Seattle 2013 y 2017. Revista Argentina de Cardiología 2019;87(2):146–51.

69. Pambo P, Adu-Adadey M, Ankrah PT, et al. Electrocardiographic and echocardiographic findings in Ghanaian female soccer players. Clin J Sport Med 2020;31(6):e367–72.

70. Gassina L-G, Jerson MN, Guessogo WR, et al. Electrocardiographic CHARACTERISTICS OF athletes OF MOUNT Cameroon ASCENT: prevention OF sudden death. Eur J Phys Education Sport Sci 2019;. https://oapub.org/edu/index.php/ejep/article/view/2243. Accessed 6 September 2022.

71. Sokunbi OJ, Okoromah CA, Ekure EN, et al. Electrocardiographic pattern of apparently healthy African adolescent athletes in Nigeria. BMC Pediatr 2021;21(1):1–12.

72. Riding NR, Sharma S, McClean G, et al. Impact of geographical origin upon the electrical and structural manifestations of the black athlete's heart. Eur Heart J 2019;40(1):50–8.

73. Pambo P, Adu-Adadey M, Agbodzakey H, et al. Electrocardiographic and echocardiographic findings in elite Ghanaian male soccer players. Clin J Sport Med 2019;31(6):e373–9.

74. Brosnan M, La Gerche A, Kumar S, et al. Modest agreement in ECG interpretation limits the application of ECG screening in young athletes. Heart Rhythm 2015;12(1):130–6.

75. Drezner JA, Asif IM, Owens DS, et al. Accuracy of ECG interpretation in competitive athletes: the impact of using standardised ECG criteria. Br J Sports Med 2012;46(5):335–40.

76. Hill AC, Miyake CY, Grady S, et al. Accuracy of interpretation of preparticipation screening electrocardiograms. J Pediatr 2011;159(5):783–8.

77. Dhutia H, Malhotra A, Yeo TJ, et al. Inter-rater reliability and downstream financial implications of electrocardiography screening in young athletes. Circ Cardiovasc Qual Outcomes 2017;10(8):e003306.

78. Calore C, Zorzi A, Sheikh N, et al. Electrocardiographic anterior T-wave inversion in athletes of different ethnicities: differential diagnosis between athlete's heart and cardiomyopathy. Eur Heart J 2015;37(32):2515–27.

79. McClean G, Riding NR, Pieles G, et al. Prevalence and significance of T-wave inversion in Arab and Black paediatric athletes: should anterior T-wave inversion interpretation be governed by biological or chronological age? Eur J Prev Cardiol 2019;26(6):641–52.

80. Petek BJ, Wasfy MM. Cardiac Adaption to exercise training: the female athlete. Curr Treat Options Cardiovasc Med 2018;20(8):68.

81. Finocchiaro G, Dhutia H, D'Silva A, et al. Effect of sex and sporting discipline on LV Adaptation to exercise. JACC: Cardiovasc Imaging 2017;10(9):965–72.

82. Malhotra A, Dhutia H, Gati S, et al. Anterior T-wave inversion in young white athletes and Nonathletes. Prevalence and Significance 2017;69(1):1–9.

83. D'Ascenzi F, Biella F, Lemme E, et al. Female athlete's heart: sex effects on electrical and structural remodeling. Circ Cardiovasc Imaging 2020;13(12):e011587.

84. Madias JE. Low QRS voltage and its causes. J Electrocardiol 2008;41(6):498–500.

85. Corrado D, van Tintelen PJ, McKenna WJ, et al. Arrhythmogenic right ventricular cardiomyopathy: evaluation of the current diagnostic criteria and differential diagnosis. Eur Heart J 2019;41(14):1414–29.

86. Caforio ALP, Pankuweit S, Arbustini E, et al. Current state of knowledge on aetiology, diagnosis, management, and therapy of myocarditis: a position statement of the European Society of Cardiology Working Group on Myocardial and Pericardial Diseases. Eur Heart J 2013;34(33):2636–48.

87. Finocchiaro G, Papadakis M, Dhutia H, et al. Electrocardiographic differentiation between 'benign T-wave inversion' and arrhythmogenic right ventricular cardiomyopathy. EP Europace 2018;21(2):332–8.

88. Brosnan MJ, Te Riele A, Bosman LP, et al. Electrocardiographic features differentiating arrhythmogenic right ventricular cardiomyopathy from an athlete's heart. JACC Clin Electrophysiol 2018;4(12):1613–25.

89. Mango F, Caselli S, Luchetti A, et al. Low QRS voltages in Olympic athletes: prevalence and clinical correlates. Eur J Prev Cardiol 2020;27(14):1542–8.

90. Zorzi A, Bettella N, Tatangelo M, et al. Prevalence and clinical significance of isolated low QRS

voltages in young athletes. Europace 2022; euab330. https://doi.org/10.1093/europace/euab330.

91. Ferreira VM, Schulz-Menger J, Holmvang G, et al. Cardiovascular magnetic resonance in nonischemic myocardial Inflammation: expert recommendations. J Am Coll Cardiol 2018;72(24):3158–76.

92. Pietrasik G, Zaręba W. QRS fragmentation: diagnostic and prognostic significance. Cardiol J 2012;19(2):114–21.

93. Das MK, Suradi H, Maskoun W, et al. Fragmented wide QRS on a 12-lead ECG. Circ Arrhythmia Electrophysiol 2008;1(4):258–68.

94. Das MK, Maskoun W, Shen C, et al. Fragmented QRS on twelve-lead electrocardiogram predicts arrhythmic events in patients with ischemic and nonischemic cardiomyopathy. Heart rhythm 2010; 7(1):74–80.

95. Peters S, Trümmel M, Koehler B. QRS fragmentation in standard ECG as a diagnostic marker of arrhythmogenic right ventricular dysplasia–cardiomyopathy. Heart Rhythm 2008;5(10): 1417–21.

96. Homsi M, Alsayed L, Safadi B, et al. Fragmented QRS complexes on 12-lead ECG: a marker of cardiac sarcoidosis as detected by gadolinium cardiac magnetic resonance imaging. Ann Noninvasive Electrocardiol 2009;14(4):319–26.

97. Morita H, Kusano KF, Miura D, et al. Fragmented QRS as a marker of conduction abnormality and a predictor of prognosis of Brugada syndrome. Circulation 2008;118(17):1697–704.

98. Corrado D, Perazzolo Marra M, Zorzi A, et al. Diagnosis of arrhythmogenic cardiomyopathy: the Padua criteria. Int J Cardiol 2020;319:106–14.

99. Marcus FI, McKenna WJ, Sherrill D, et al. Diagnosis of arrhythmogenic right ventricular cardiomyopathy/dysplasia: proposed modification of the task force criteria. Eur Heart J 2010;31(7):806–14.

100. Ollitrault P, Pellissier A, Champ-Rigot L, et al. Prevalence and significance of fragmented QRS complex in lead V1 on the surface electrocardiogram of healthy athletes. EP Europace 2020;22(4): 649–56.

101. Zorzi A, Vio R, Bettella N, et al. Criteria for interpretation of the athlete's ECG: a critical appraisal. Pacing Clin Electrophysiol 2020;43(8):882–90.

102. Corrado D, Drezner JA, D'Ascenzi F, et al. How to evaluate premature ventricular beats in the athlete: critical review and proposal of a diagnostic algorithm. Br J Sports Med 2020;54(19):1142–8.

103. Palatini P, Maraglino G, Sperti G, et al. Prevalence and possible mechanisms of ventricular arrhythmias in athletes. Am Heart J 1985;110(3):560–7.

104. Talan DA, Bauernfeind RA, Ashley WW, et al. Twenty-four hour continuous ECG recordings in long-distance runners. Chest 1982;82(1):19–24.

105. Viitasalo M, Kala R, Eisalo A. Ambulatory electrocardiographic recording in endurance athletes. Heart 1982;47(3):213–20.

106. Viitasalo M, Kala R, Eisalo A. Ambulatory electrocardiographic findings in young athletes between 14 and 16 years of age. Eur Heart J 1984;5(1):2–6.

107. Zorzi A, De Lazzari M, Mastella G, et al. Ventricular arrhythmias in young competitive athletes: prevalence, determinants, and underlying substrate. J Am Heart Assoc 2018;7(12):e009171.

108. Pilcher GF, Cook AJ, Johnston BL, et al. Twenty-four-hour continuous electrocardiography during exercise and free activity in 80 apparently healthy runners. Am J Cardiol 1983;52(7):859–61.

109. Haghjoo M, Mohammadzadeh S, Taherpour M, et al. ST-segment depression as a risk factor in hypertrophic cardiomyopathy. EP Europace 2009; 11(5):643–9.

110. Maron BJ, Wolfson JK, Ciró E, et al. Relation of electrocardiographic abnormalities and patterns of left ventricular hypertrophy identified by 2-dimensional echocardiography in patients with hypertrophic cardiomyopathy. Am J Cardiol 1983; 51(1):189–94.

111. Kim JH, Noseworthy PA, McCarty D, et al. Significance of electrocardiographic right bundle branch block in trained athletes. Am J Cardiol 2011;107(7): 1083–9.

112. Kim JH, Baggish AL. Electrocardiographic right and left bundle branch block patterns in athletes: prevalence, pathology, and clinical significance. J Electrocardiol 2015;48(3):380–4.

Anomalous Coronary Arteries
A State-of-the-Art Approach

Silvana Molossi, MD, PhD[a,b],*, Tam Doan, MD[a,b], Shagun Sachdeva, MD[a,b]

KEYWORDS

- Sudden cardiac death • Anomalous aortic origin of a coronary artery • Coronary artery anomalies
- Advanced imaging • Cardiac catheterization

KEY POINTS

- Congenital anomalies of the coronary arteries may affect up to 1% of the population and lead to myocardial ischemia and sudden death.
- Echocardiography can diagnose anomalous coronaries in up to 95% of patients, though advanced imaging has greatly enhanced the ability to define morphologic features that impact outcome.
- Risk stratification remains a challenge in the setting of anomalous aortic origin of a coronary artery (AAOCA), and myocardial functional studies under provocative stress greatly contribute to management decision-making.
- Standardized approach to the evaluation and management of patients with coronary anomalies, with data gathering and collaboration among institutions, are paramount to optimize outcomes in this population.
- Optimal strategies in management will foster a safer environment for patients with coronary anomalies to engage in exercise and sports participation, essential components to successful and healthier lives.

INTRODUCTION

Congenital anomalies of the coronary arteries represent a varied group of lesions and are seen in less than 1% to 5% of the population, depending on method of diagnosis.[1,2] Embryologic development of the coronary artery is not completely understood, although altered coronary embryogenesis may result in abnormal coronary origins from the aorta or pulmonary artery or incomplete development leading to coronary fistulae or sinusoids. It can occur as an isolated anomaly or in association with other congenital heart diseases. Although many coronary artery anomalies are detected as incidental findings with little to no significant consequence, approximately 20% of all may have a potential risk of coronary ischemia leading to myocardial infarction, arrhythmia, and sudden cardiac death (SCD).[1-3] This report focuses on the anatomy, physiology, diagnostic strategy, and management of isolated anomalous origin of a coronary artery from the aorta and from the pulmonary artery.

ANOMALOUS AORTIC ORIGIN OF A CORONARY ARTERY
Prevalence and Clinical Significance

The true prevalence of anomalous aortic origin of a coronary artery (AAOCA) in the general population remains unknown because studies have focused primarily on symptomatic patients. The estimated frequency of anomalous aortic origin of the left

[a] Coronary Artery Anomalies Program, Texas Children's Hospital, 6651 Main Street, MC E1920, Houston, TX 77030, USA; [b] The Lillie Frank Abercrombie Section of Cardiology, Texas Children's Hospital, Baylor College of Medicine, 6651 Main Street, MC E1920, Houston, TX 77030, USA
* Corresponding author. Coronary Artery Anomalies Program, Texas Children's Hospital, 6651 Main Street, MC E1920, Houston, TX 77030.
E-mail address: smolossi@bcm.edu

Cardiol Clin 41 (2023) 51–69
https://doi.org/10.1016/j.ccl.2022.08.005
0733-8651/23/© 2022 Elsevier Inc. All rights reserved.

coronary artery (AAOLCA) is 0.03% to 0.15%, whereas that of anomalous aortic origin of the right coronary artery (AAORCA) is 0.28% to 0.92%.[1,4] AAOCA is known to be the second leading cause of SCD in young athletes, estimated to be responsible for 15% to 20% of sudden death in this population.[3,5] The risk of SCD seems highest in young individuals, particularly during or following a period of strenuous exertion, and particularly in those with interarterial and intramural AAOLCA. Studies of adult cohorts with AAORCA undergoing conservative therapy have observed a very low mortality (<1%) in about 1 to 5 years of follow-up.[4,6]

Anatomic subtypes and pathophysiology

This anomaly can involve either the right coronary originating from the left sinus of Valsalva (reportedly more common) or the left coronary originating from the right sinus of Valsalva (**Fig. 1**), and rarely more posteriorly from the noncoronary sinus or near the posterior commissure with or without an intramural course.[7]

Several pathophysiologic mechanisms have been postulated for the occurrence of sudden cardiac arrest (SCA)/SCD in patients with AAOCA. These include occlusion and/or compression of the anomalous coronary artery (intramural segment, interarterial course) and ostial abnormalities (slit-like and stenotic ostium), particularly during exercise, leading to myocardial ischemia and development of ventricular arrhythmia.[8] In a study by Basso and colleagues, of 27 individuals who experienced SCD due to AAOCA, only 10 presented with symptoms before the event.[5] Given the significant number of patients that are asymptomatic before a critical adverse cardiac event, this highlights difficulties in evaluating patients at risk for adverse sudden cardiac events.

Clinical evaluation

Clinical Presentation and Diagnosis

In recent studies, about 50% of patients have been noted to be asymptomatic at diagnosis.[3,8–12] An increasing number of children and adolescents are being diagnosed with AAOCA following routine preparticipation screening, presence of a murmur, or an abnormal electrocardiogram (ECG).[10,11] Typical presenting symptoms that have been reported are exertional chest pain, palpitations, syncope, as well as SCA.[11,12]

Transthoracic echocardiography (TTE) is the first-line imaging modality for the initial diagnosis.[13,14] Recent report by Lorber and colleagues, found variable agreement between TTE and surgical findings.[14] In another study, TTE reliably and prospectively diagnosed AAOCA in more than 95% of the cohort, and the echo findings were always consistent with the surgical descriptions of the anatomy.[10] Lorber and colleagues also suggested that, apart from the use of TTE in the diagnosis of the abnormal coronary origins, TTE can be helpful in identifying critical anatomic features such as intramural/interarterial course, which may influence surgical management. However, they demonstrated that the assessment of coronary ostium as well as intramyocardial course was not well delineated by TTE. Thus, advanced imaging modalities, including computed tomography angiography (CTA) or cardiac magnetic resonance imaging (CMR) are extremely helpful in comprehensively defining the anatomy of the AAOCA, including ostial morphology, interarterial, intramural, or intramyocardial course.[15–22]

Noninvasive Testing Under Provocative Stress

Exercise stress test Exercise stress test (EST) is recommended in the evaluation of patients with coronary anomalies to assess for ischemic changes during exercise.[23,24] It has been used widely in children with coronary artery anomalies who can tolerate exercise, although it has a low sensitivity to detect inducible ischemia in this population.[5,10,23–29] Moreover, the interpretation of inducible ischemia may vary according to different studies when EST is reported "abnormal," which may reflect blunted blood pressure response, occurrence of premature ventricular contractions, or ST segment depression/elevation, the latter clearly with high specificity indicating inducible myocardial ischemia.[10,22,27,30] SCD during exertion has been reported in patients with coronary artery anomalies who had a normal EST before the event.[5] Brothers and colleagues reported a patient with AAOCA who initially had ischemic changes on EST but a repeat EST 1 week later was reassuring, which raised the question of intermittent nature of ischemia in the setting of AAOCA.[31] Current guidelines state that asymptomatic patients with AAORCA would be considered low-risk if EST is normal.[23,24] However, compelling data by Qasim and colleagues demonstrated the addition of cardiopulmonary exercise testing improved sensitivity of EST in patients with AAOCA, although EST is not well correlated with dobutamine stress CMR (DSCMR; **Fig. 2**).[26] Additionally, ischemic changes were recorded in only 1% of EST in a group of 164 patients with AAORCA.[25] Despite having a poor sensitivity, EST remains a valuable tool and seems to be specific in the presence of ST segment changes suggestive of myocardial ischemia. Continued data gathering and correlation with other provocative

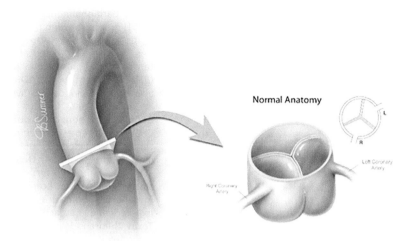

Normal Anatomy

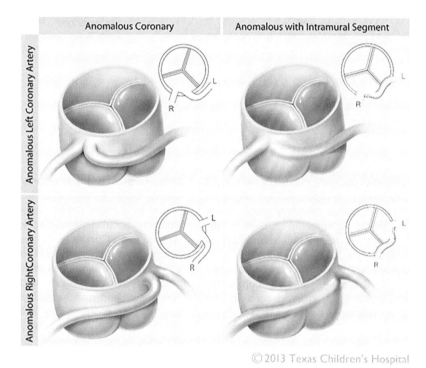

Anomalous Coronary   Anomalous with Intramural Segment

Anomalous Left Coronary Artery

Anomalous RightCoronary Artery

© 2013 Texas Children's Hospital

Fig. 1. Normal coronary anatomy and AAOCA subtypes. Used with permission of Texas Children's Hospital.

tests investigating inducible myocardial ischemia is needed to further define its role in this young population with AAOCA.

Stress echocardiography Stress echocardiography has been established to identify new regional wall motion abnormalities or valvular dysfunction indicative of inducible myocardial ischemia following exercise (treadmill/cycloergometer) or during pharmacologic stress using dobutamine/atropine or adenosine/dipyridimole.[32–38] Heart rate decreases quickly, particularly in young children, a limitation that may prevent accurate acquisition and reading of images. Pharmacologic stimuli, however, allow for sustained peak heart rate with optimal image acquisition during peak stress, including in smaller children or infants.[39] It is available in most centers, portable, and less expensive than other advanced imaging modalities. Notwithstanding, training and expertise is important in the assessment of regional wall motion abnormalities, which may limit its use in centers with low patient volume and/or with variable readers. Yet, stress echocardiography has been

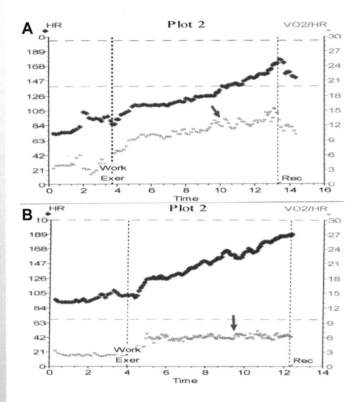

Fig. 2. Cardiopulmonary exercise testing (CPET) graphs showing normal upsloping O_2 pulse curve (*blue arrow*) (*A*) in a patient with AAORCA and abnormal flattening of O_2 pulse curve (*blue arrow*) (*B*) in a patient with AAORCA (patient also had subendocardial hypoperfusion in anterior and inferior septum on DSCMR). The horizontal dotted line on CPET graphs represents the maximal percentage predicted O_2 pulse for body mass. (*From* Qasim A, Doan TT, Pham TDN, Molossi S. Poster: Exercise stress testing in risk stratification of Anomalous Aortic Origin of a Coronary Artery. In: Pediatric Reseacrh Symposium at Texas Children's Hospital. ; 2021. https://www.texaschildrens.org/sites/default/files/uploads/documents/symposia/2021/posters/90.pdf. Printed with permission from Texas Children's Hospital.)

used in the pediatric population with a wide variety of indications where coronary lesions are suspected, such as acquired coronary disease and repaired/unrepaired congenital heart disease,[34,35,40,41] and as the preferred method to evaluate inducible myocardial ischemia in children/adolescents with AAOCA in some centers.[10,22,39,42–44] Currently, studies comparing different noninvasive testing modalities in the assessment of myocardial perfusion in AAOCA is lacking.

Advanced imaging on provocative stress
Nuclear perfusion imaging Nuclear perfusion imaging (NPI) with provocative stress is well established in adults for the evaluation of coronary artery/ischemic heart disease. Its use in the evaluation of inducible ischemia in the young with AAOCA has been reported by several groups (**Fig. 3**B).[22,27,30,44–47] However, concerns with patient exposure to ionizing radiation, high incidence of false-positive and false-negative findings, low spatial resolution, and attenuation artifacts are all factors that have resulted in decreasing interest for the use of NPI in this population. These are reasons that led our institution to transition to DSCMR as its safety, feasibility, and utility in a large cohort of children and adolescents with AAOCA have been recently published.[27,28,48–50]

Stress cardiac magnetic resonance imaging Stress cardiac magnetic resonance imaging has been reported to improve patient outcome when used to guide revascularization decision in adults with ischemic heart disease.[51–60] Several studies have demonstrated its safety and feasibility in children with coronary artery involvement following a diagnosis of Kawasaki disease and repaired complex congenital heart disease that include coronary artery transfer (ie, following arterial switch operation).[61–65] In these studies, hyperemia was achieved using adenosine or its selective alpha-2A receptor agonist (Regadenoson) to potentially unmask fixed obstructive coronary lesions. The proposed mechanism by which inducible ischemia may occur in patients with AAOCA has been postulated to relate to dynamic obstruction during exertion, although ostial abnormalities may be contributory as a fixed mechanism. Dobutamine has been viewed to closely mimic exercise because it increases contractility and decreases systemic vascular resistance,[56,57,65,66] thus inducing wall motion abnormalities at a time of maximal myocardial oxygen demand. DSCMR has demonstrated excellent performance with good prediction of ischemic events in adults.[54,66,67] First-pass perfusion, in addition to assessment of wall motion abnormalities, has increased the sensitivity of DSCMR, in keeping with the mechanism in demand ischemia cascade

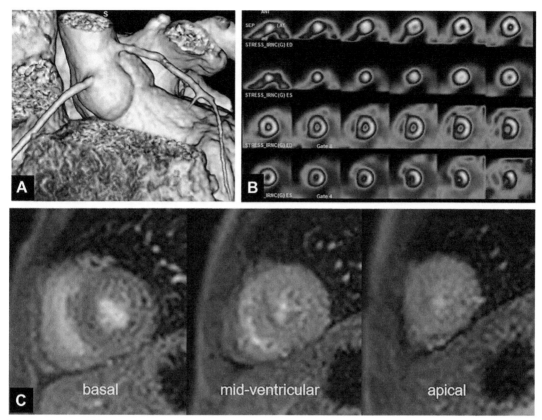

Fig. 3. A 9-year-old boy with AAOLCA at the sinotubular junction near the intercoronary commissure on CTA (*A*). Patient had a reassuring nuclear stress perfusion study (*B*), and no subendocardial hypoperfusion on DSCMR (*C*).

(where impaired perfusion precedes wall motion abnormalities).[56–58,60] Stress CMR additionally provides high-quality cardiac imaging with excellent spatial resolution and avoids ionizing radiation, an important factor especially in children/adolescents.[68–71] Doan and colleagues reported the largest cohort of children with AAOCA undergoing DSCMR,[48] including 224 studies in 182 patients younger than 20 years and median age of 14 years. Most studies were successfully completed with no sedation and 99% were free of major events, with only 12.5% reported minor events (**Fig. 3**; **Fig. 4**). Inducible perfusion defects were seen in 14%, and 42% among these had associated wall motion abnormalities. This study demonstrated safety and feasibility of DSCMR in the young patient with AAOCA and greatly contributed to management decisions.[48] Moreover, agreement between DSCMR and invasive fractional flow reserve (FFR) during dobutamine challenge was demonstrated in 13 young patients with AAOCA.[72] Comparable data was demonstrated in isolated case reports and intraseptal AAOLCA in a cohort of 19 patients reported by Doan and colleagues.[73–75] These authors

reported stress perfusion imaging studies in 14 patients and 50% had inducible perfusion defects.[75] Given these more recent data, DSCMR clearly seems to have a defining role for the detection of perfusion abnormalities in AAOCA, allowing for comparison of results after surgical repair (in those patients for whom this intervention is indicated) with resolution of the inducible ischemia determined postoperatively (see **Fig. 4**).[27,28,48,49] However, image quality and expertise are paramount for the visual assessment of first-pass perfusion of gadolinium, specifically to differentiate dark rim artifacts from a true inducible perfusion defect. Risk stratification in AAOCA continues to be a challenge to determine those patients at risk for myocardial ischemia and DSCMR is clearly contributing to decision-making in this population.

Invasive Testing Under Provocative Stress

Angiography Angiography is generally not the first choice of imaging to diagnose anomalous coronary arteries in children. However, it is part of invasive assessment of coronary artery flow and has been performed in recent years when there is

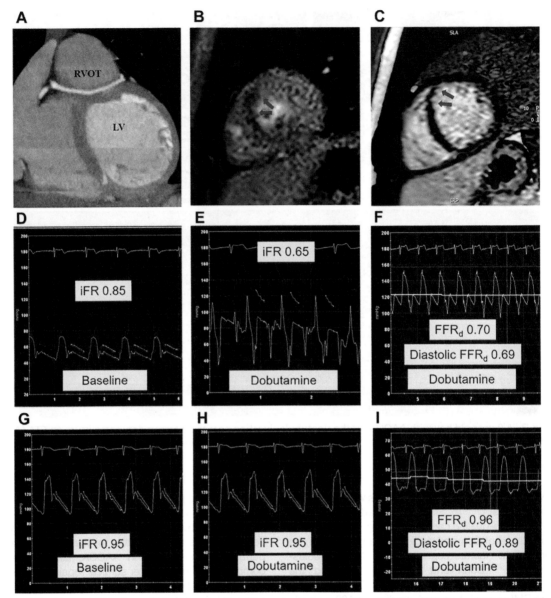

Fig. 4. A 16-year-old male patient with recurrent chest pain during wrestling practice. CTA showed AAOLCA with intraseptal course of the LCA (*A*). DSCMR showed subendocardial hypoperfusion in the anteroseptal wall (*red arrows*) (*B*), and late-gadolinium enhancement (*red arrows*) (*C*) indicates inducible ischemia and likely history of subendocardial infarction. Baseline iFR <0.89 (*D*), which further decreased to 0.65 (*E*), and diastolic FFR 0.69 <0.80 (*F*) consistent with impaired coronary flow. Following supraarterial myotomy of the intraseptal segment through a right ventriculotomy and direct reimplantation of the LCA, there were normalization of baseline iFR to 0.95 (*G*); at peak dobutamine stress, normal values of iFR at 0.95 (*H*), FFR at 0.96, and diastolic FFR at 0.89 (*I*). (*From* Doan TT, Molossi S, Qureshi AM, McKenzie ED. Intraseptal Anomalous Coronary Artery With Myocardial Infarction: Novel Surgical Approach. Ann Thorac Surg. 2020 Oct;110(4):e271-e274.)

conflict between clinical data and results from noninvasive studies.[76,77] Using pharmacologic stressors to mimic physiologic changes that occur during exercise may disclose hemodynamically significant lesions that would benefit from intervention, including measurement of coronary flow and angiographic assessment of the vessel diameter (**Fig. 5**B, C).

Fractional flow reserve FFR is a pressure-derived index of severity in the setting of coronary artery stenosis, calculated as a ratio between mean

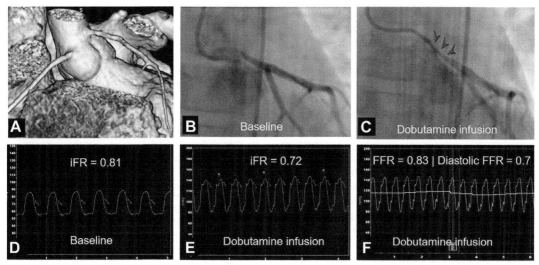

Fig. 5. Angiogram and intracoronary hemodynamic assessment in a 9-year-old boy with AAOLCA at the sinotubular junction near the intercoronary commissure on CTA (*A*). Despite reassuring DSCMR and nuclear stress perfusion study (see **Fig. 3**), the proximal LCA caliber changed from subtle narrowing (*B*) to severely compressed (*red arrowheads*) during dobutamine infusion (*C*). Baseline iFR <0.89 indicates significant coronary artery compression (*D*) and iFR further reduced during dobutamine infusion (*E*). Diastolic FFR <0.8 consistent with significant coronary flow impairment during provocative testing with dobutamine (*F*).

intracoronary pressure distal to the lesion (Pd) and mean aortic pressure (Pa) obtained during the entire cardiac cycle (see **Fig. 4**; **Fig. 5**). It requires the use of a coronary vasodilator to unmask a fixed obstructive coronary lesion. In adults with ischemic heart disease, coronary revascularization is typically indicated with FFR less than 0.8. In the setting of dynamic mechanisms leading to coronary compression, such as in AAOCA with intramural course or intraseptal course, dobutamine is considered the preferred pharmacologic agent to induce provocative stress mimicking some physiologic changes that occur with exercise.[48,65,78] Dobutamine induces positive inotropy and increased cardiac output, as it also induces decrease in systemic and coronary vascular resistance.[79–81] Diastolic FFR (dFFR), however, might constitute a better indicator of intracoronary hemodynamic assessment during dobutamine infusion given a potential overshooting of distal systolic pressure, which in turn may nullify a significant diastolic pressure gradient.[82] The initial data on the use of FFR in children with AAOCA was presented by Agrawal and colleagues in 2017, although in a small cohort that included 4 patients with AAOCA, stating its contribution in risk stratification in select patients.[76] As dFFR is calculated manually (average of 3 Pd/Pa ratio using digital calipers at end systole), it comprises a major limitation. In addition, the use of dobutamine is contraindicated in

patients presenting with SCA, further limiting the assessment of FFR in AAOCA.

Instantaneous wave-free ratio Instantaneous wave-free ratio (iFR) is a drug-free pressure-derived index of coronary artery flow during a period of naturally constant and low resistance due to minimal competing pressure waves in diastole (see **Figs. 4** and **5**).[83] In theory, advantages of this index include no need of a vasodilator to reduce coronary vascular resistance and better procedure tolerance due to shorter procedure time.[84] iFR showed better agreement with coronary flow velocity reserve when compared with (JUSTIFY-CFR study)[85] and noninferior to FFR because it relates to health outcomes in guiding coronary revascularization in adults with ischemic heart disease.[84,86] Doan and colleagues very recently first reported the use of iFR in children with AAOCA.[78] Data showed that iFR correlated with adenosine FFR and dobutamine dFFR, thus being an alternative to those patients in which pharmacologic stressors (eg, dobutamine) are contraindicated. Moreover, the authors stated the data contributed to decision-making regarding coronary intervention. Additional recent data from the same authors published resting iFR and dFFR with dobutamine challenge guiding decision-making in a subset of patients with concerning clinical symptoms but negative noninvasive perfusion studies under provocative stress.[87] These abnormal values of intracoronary flow were shown to completely resolve on repeat invasive studies following surgical intervention (see **Fig. 4**G–I).

Of interest, the principles of iFR during dobutamine challenge neutralizes the systolic overshooting phenomenon in the assessment of potential dynamic compression in AAOCA, indicating that dynamic compression during provocative stress could be of value in unfolding hemodynamic significant coronary obstruction in the setting of AAOCA. Specifically, Ghobrial and colleagues published their center experience in symptomatic adult AAOCA patients using iFR and dobutamine challenge.[88] Similarly, these authors reported improvement in dobutamine iFR in 18 patients following surgical repair of the anomalous vessel. We have observed similar pattern of provocative pharmacologic stress with dobutamine affect iFR values in children with AAOCA compared with those seen at rest in our center (unpublished data). As promising as these data on significant improvement in iFR and FFR following surgical repair of AAOCA are,[89] it is important to keep in perspective that such cutoff values derive from ischemic coronary artery disease in adults and may not be the optimal values in the setting of AAOCA, which likely includes mostly a dynamic component leading to myocardial ischemia and sudden events, especially in the young population.

Intravascular ultrasound Intravascular ultrasound (IVUS) in AAOCA has been widely used in adults and considered the gold standard for the assessment of the intramural segment given its excellent spatial determination and evaluation of dynamic lateral compression at rest and compared with pharmacologic stress.[4,90–92] Angelini and colleagues published data in adult patients with AAORCA where IVUS showed the worst area of stenosis in the intramural segment of the RCA proximally, immediately distal to its ostium.[90] IVUS performed under pharmacologic stress includes administration of saline bolus, atropine, and dobutamine. The diameter (minimal and maximal) of the anomalous coronary in the compromised area is measured in both systole and diastole. Significant coronary compression includes an area ratio greater than 50% at baseline and/or greater than 60% during provocative stress.[90] Its use has also guided stent placement in the proximal intramural segment in select adults patients with AAORCA.[90] Although IVUS is used in pediatric patients for the evaluation of certain congenital heart lesions,[93] its use in the setting of AAOCA is hardly existent. Agrawal and colleagues reported a small cohort of pediatric patients with AAOCA and myocardial

bridges describing the feasibility and safety of IVUS, and its significant contribution in management decision-making.[76] This seems promising in a very selected group of patients with AAOCA but substantial data are needed to determine its role in risk stratification in young patients. More importantly, perhaps, this should not be considered a common technique in the evaluation of young patients with AAOCA because expertise is essential to mitigate potential serious coronary complications with the procedure.

Management decision-making

Medical Management

At our institution, we use a previously published standardized approach in the assessment and management of AAOCA (**Fig. 6**).[27] Clinical follow-up without medication or intervention is indicated when the provocative testing is negative for ischemic changes in the asymptomatic patient with AAORCA.[94] Exercise restriction with or without beta-blocker therapy (in the setting of intraseptal AAOLCA) is indicated when surgery is recommended in a patient with AAOCA but surgery is either denied or not feasible given the anatomy.[73] In our experience, medical management in a young athlete with beta-blocker therapy is challenging given its effect in athletic performance. Therefore, surgical intervention is favored when it outweighs the risks. Following surgical repair of the anomalous coronary artery, we empirically recommend antiplatelet therapy with aspirin for 3 months, with discontinuation following reassuring postoperative studies at this time.

Surgical Approach

To date, the exact mechanisms of ischemia leading to SCA in AAOCA remain undefined, as do clinical and morphologic features that increase the risk of ischemia and SCA.[95–98] Surgical repair of AAOCA has been performed to potentially address this risk and mitigate the occurrence of SCA, although surgical indications and benefits remain unclear with significant variation in practice.[10,12,28,49,99,100] Current consensus guidelines provide a standardized approach that surgical intervention is recommended for those with signs and/or symptoms of ischemia (class I).[23,24,94] In asymptomatic patients with reassuring diagnostic testing, surgery is recommended (class IIa) for patients with AAORCA who had ventricular arrhythmia and in AAOLCA.[94] Patients who are diagnosed with AAORCA can be considered for surgery despite reassuring testing and no other clinical concern (class IIb).[94] The goals of AAOCA repair are to yield an unobstructed coronary artery from the appropriate aortic sinus while minimizing the risk of procedural complications.[28,101] Surgical

Clinical algorithm for patients with anomalous aortic origin or course of a coronary artery

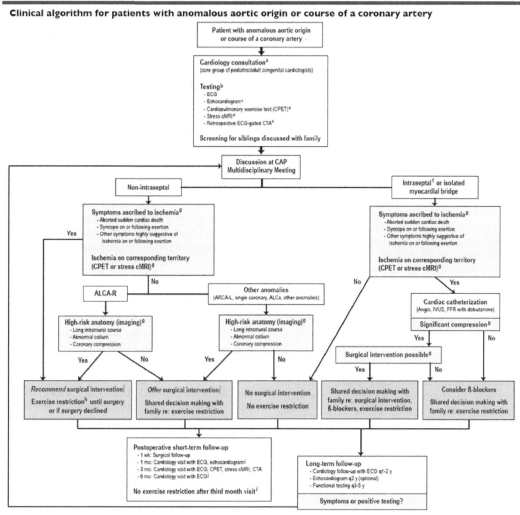

Fig. 6. Clinical algorithm for patients with anomalous aortic origin of a coronary artery. ALCA-R, anomalous left coronary from the right sinus; ALCx, anomalous left circumflex artery; ARCA-L, anomalous right coronary from the left sinus; CAP, coronary anomalies program. [a]Consent abtained for participation in prospective CHSS aand TCH databases. [b]Additional studies (Holter, cardiac catheterization, etc) may be performed depending on the clinical assessment. [c]External echocardiograms do not need to be repeated if the study is deemed appropriate. [d]CPET or stress cMRI not necessary on patients that present with aborted sudden cardiac death. These studies may be deferred in young patients. [e]An external CTA may be used if able to upload the images and the study provides all necessary information to make a decision. CTA should ne deferred in patients <8 years unless clinical concerns. [f]An intraseptal coronaru is as an abnormal vessel(usually a left coronary arising from the right sinus)that travels posteriorly into the septum below the level of the pulmonary valve. [g]Unrollfing if significant intramural segment, neo-ostium creation or voronary translocation if intramural segment behind a commissure, coronary translocation if short or no intramural segment. Surgical intervention will be offered for patients between 10 and 35 years of age. Other patients will be considered on a case-by-case basis. Aspirin will be administered for 3 months after surgery. [h]Restriction form participation in all competitive sports and in exercise with moderate or high dynamic component(> 40% maximal oxygen uptake-e.g., soccer, tennis, swimming, basketball, American football). (Mitchell et al, JACC 2005:1364-1367). [i]Patient may be seen by outside primary cardiologist. [j]Postoperative patients will be cleared for exercise and competitive sports based on findings at the third month postoperative visit including results of CPET, stress cMRI and CTA. Used with permission of Texas Children's Hospital.

repair of AAOCA should aim at eliminating the intramural course and its associated ostial narrowing by unroofing, ostioplasty, or transection and reimplantation (TAR).[24] Unroofing of an intramural course is most commonly reported, although other techniques including TAR or neo-ostium creation have also been performed.[10,28,49,99,102,103] Repositioning of the pulmonary artery confluence away from the

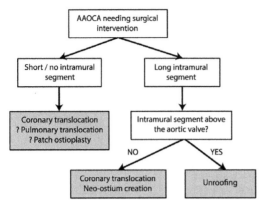

Fig. 7. Proposed algorithm to select surgical intervention techniques for patients with AAOCA based on coronary artery anatomy using computerized tomography angiography and surgical inspection. (*From* Mery CM, De León LE, Molossi S, Sexson-Tejtel SK, Agrawal H, Krishnamurthy R, Masand P, Qureshi AM, McKenzie ED, Fraser CD Jr. Outcomes of surgical intervention for anomalous aortic origin of a coronary artery: A large contemporary prospective cohort study. J Thorac Cardiovasc Surg. 2018 Jan;155(1):305-319.e4.)

anomalous artery may be considered as an adjunctive procedure but less widely used.[24] Surgical intervention is generally successful, although complication and reoperation due to coronary artery stenosis have been reported up to 5% in the 7 years following the index operation in a multicenter study.[99]

Anomalous aortic origin of a coronary artery with interarterial course or anomalous aortic origin of the left coronary artery from the noncoronary sinus The primary surgical strategies described at our center included unroofing of an intramural course and coronary TAR (**Fig. 7**). We do not favor takedown of the aortic commissure at the time of surgical unroofing due to the potential risk of postoperative aortic insufficiency.[28] Unroofing has been our surgical procedure of choice for patients with an intramural segment above the aortic valve in which the technique is believed to move the ostium to the correct sinus. TAR has been used for patients with short intramural length and the intramural segment traveling below the level of the aortic valve commissure, in whom surgical unroofing would not result in placing the ostium in its correct aortic sinus (**Fig. 8**).[28,49,101]

Coronary unroofing is a widely used technique and is considered relatively safe in the surgical repair of AAOCA.[10,103–106] Coronary TAR has been performed in both adults and children when the unroofing technique is deemed to have potential disruption of the aortic valve integrity.[49,100,107,108] TAR requires

extensive coronary manipulation involving transection followed by reimplantation of the anomalous coronary artery without an aortic button. It is important to emphasize that it is still unknown which surgical technique is superior, and that TAR should only be considered in select candidates and performed in centers with expertise given the technical complexity with potential iatrogenic complications.[109]

Anomalous aortic origin of the left coronary artery with intraseptal course Surgical intervention for this anomaly is challenged by the limitation of current surgical techniques and the uncertainty of long-term outcomes. Najm and colleagues performed unroofing of the intraseptal LCA by circumferentially transecting and extending the right ventricular infundibulum using autologous pericardium.[110,111] The authors reported excellent surgical outcome in 14 patients who have been followed between 1.5 and 45 months.[111] Others have reported anterior translocation of the right pulmonary artery and division of the muscle overlying the LCA externally between the aortic root and pulmonary artery.[12] We have reported a successful supraarterial myotomy of the intraseptal segment through a right ventriculotomy and direct reimplantation of the left coronary artery. This patient recovered well with improved physiologic provocative testing following surgery and has returned to competitive wrestling without issues.[74]

Recommendations to physical activities

Consensus guidelines state that individuals with AAOCA and symptoms of ischemic chest pain or syncope suspected to be due to ventricular arrhythmias, or a history of aborted SCD, should be activity restricted and offered surgery.[24] The asymptomatic patient with AAORCA and no evidence of ischemia clinically and with provocative testing can participate in competitive athletics. However, patients and family should be appropriately informed and counseled of the known risk of SCD, although rare, and the uncertain accuracy of a negative stress test.[23] It is important to recommend preparedness for cardiac events such as having an automated external defibrillator (AED) available with individuals who know how to use it, as part of an emergency action plan. However, individuals with untreated AAOLCA from the opposite (right) anterior sinus of Valsalva, regardless of symptomatology, are restricted from all competitive sports.[23,24,94]

Following successful surgical repair of AAOCA, athletes may consider participation in all sports 3 months after surgery if the patient remains free of symptoms, an EST shows no evidence of ischemia or cardiac arrhythmias, and a stress

A Long intramural length >5 mm and the coronary courses above the commissure

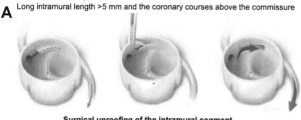

Surgical unroofing of the intramural segment

B Thickened pillar   Intramural length <5 mm   Course below the commissure

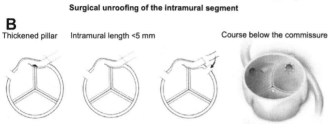

Transection and Reimplantation

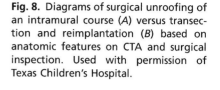

Fig. 8. Diagrams of surgical unroofing of an intramural course (*A*) versus transection and reimplantation (*B*) based on anatomic features on CTA and surgical inspection. Used with permission of Texas Children's Hospital.

perfusion imaging study shows no inducible perfusion defect or regional wall motion abnormalities.[24,27,28] In patients who presented with aborted SCD, a longer postoperative period (12 months) may be necessary to ensure patients are free of symptoms suggesting ischemia or arrhythmia and have no evidence of myocardial ischemia on provocative testing or concerning arrhythmia.[24] An AED should be available for all of these patients with available personnel who are trained in cardiopulmonary resuscitation and how to use an AED.[24]

ANOMALOUS CORONARY ARTERY ORIGIN FROM THE PULMONARY ARTERY
Prevalence, Anatomy, Physiology, and Diagnosis

Prevalence
Anomalous origin of the left coronary artery from pulmonary artery (ALCAPA) is a rare disease, occurring in 1 in 3,00,000 live births or 0.4% of patients with congenital cardiac abnormalities,[112] that if untreated causes heart failure, myocardial ischemia, and death. The incidence of ALCAPA is thought to be higher than that of anomalous origin of the right coronary artery from pulmonary artery (ARCAPA) due to the proximity of the left coronary bud to the pulmonary artery sinus (although ARCAPA may have been underdiagnosed due to its initially relatively innocuous nature compared with ALCAPA).[113,114] ARCAPA is known to occur in 0.002% of patients with congenital cardiac abnormalities.[114–116]

Anatomy
The most common defect of this type is ALCAPA, sometimes known as Bland-White-Garland

syndrome.[117,118] In some cases, the left anterior descending and left circumflex coronary arteries have individual origins from the pulmonary artery, with similar pathophysiologic and clinical sequelae.[119,120] The origin of the right coronary artery from the pulmonary artery has been thought to be benign; however, clinical sequelae have been described although later in life.[121]

Physiology
Fetuses with ALCAPA remain asymptomatic because the diastolic pressure in the pulmonary artery and aorta are similar during prenatal circulation. When the pulmonary vascular resistance starts to drop after birth, symptoms start to appear in most infants due to a reversal flow through left coronary artery. This leads to coronary artery steal and further progression of myocardial ischemia. This may be exacerbated during periods of stress, which in infants can occur during feedings. The surrounding arteries start to create collateral blood flow to the affected ventricle. Mitral valve regurgitation occurs in the disease process secondary to ventricular dilatation and papillary muscle ischemia. Patients may initially present with subtle symptoms of extreme fussiness with feeds, due to the ischemia, and ultimately progress toward respiratory distress as heart failure ensues.[122–124] Nevertheless, many patients may do well and be completely asymptomatic, engaging in sports activities until late childhood and adolescence when the diagnosis is established following evaluation for a murmur (commonly mitral regurgitation from chronic ischemia to the mitral valve apparatus).

Due to the reduced ventricular workload and oxygen demands of the right ventricle compared with that of the left ventricle, ventricular ischemia is less prominent in ARCAPA than in ALCAPA and may present in adult life. However, ARCAPA patients with a right dominant coronary circulation do exhibit chronic ischemia and have increased adverse outcomes than patients with a left dominant circulation.[125,126]

Diagnosis

This condition is usually suspected on echocardiography either by direct visualization of the coronary artery from the pulmonary artery or by secondary signs of ventricular dysfunction, mitral regurgitation, echogenic papillary muscles, dilation of right coronary artery (due to collateral formation in ALCAPA) as well as the presence of flow signals within the myocardium suggesting collateral flow (**Figs. 9** and **10**).[127,128] Noninvasive cross-sectional imaging with either CTA or CMR may assist in more definitive diagnosis and provide additional information.

The electrocardiogram of a patient with ALCAPA may show evidence for anterolateral ischemia or infarction, including transient or chronic ST-segment changes in the anterolateral leads or Q waves in leads I aVL, V5, and V6.[129]

Although patients with ARCAPA may mirror the symptoms of ALCAPA, it is usually diagnosed at autopsy or in asymptomatic children or adults. Electrocardiographic findings are often nonspecific. The diagnosis can be made with careful TTE that includes meticulous attention to the origins of the coronary arteries. CTA of the coronary arteries is also diagnostic. Alternatively, cardiac catheterization provides hemodynamic assessment in addition to coronary angiography to confirm the diagnosis.[114,116,130]

Surgical Approach

All anomalously originating coronary arteries from the pulmonary artery require surgical correction. At this time, there are no percutaneous treatment options to repair this anomaly.

Anomalous origin of the left coronary artery from the pulmonary artery

Regardless of clinical status, patients with ALCAPA would require urgent operation.[130] Creating a two-artery coronary system is indicated in all situations, including critically ill infants. Available pathologic information indicates that either a tunnel (Takeuchi)

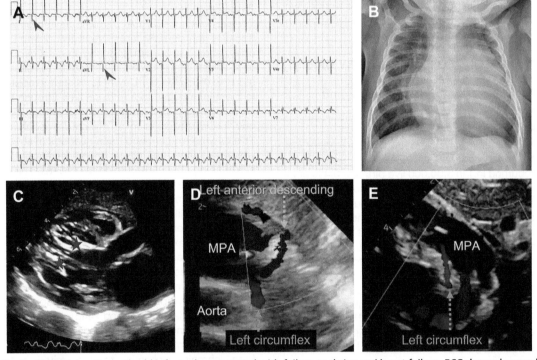

Fig. 9. ALCAPA in a 2-month-old infant who presented with failure to thrive and heart failure. ECG showed normal sinus rhythm, left axis deviation, Q wave in lead I and aVL (*arrowheads*), and T-wave inversion in the inferolateral leads (*A*), severe cardiomegaly and pulmonary edema (*B*), echogenic papillary muscles (*red stars*, C), retrograde flow in the left anterior descending coronary artery (*D*), and circumflex artery (*E*). MPA, main pulmonary artery.

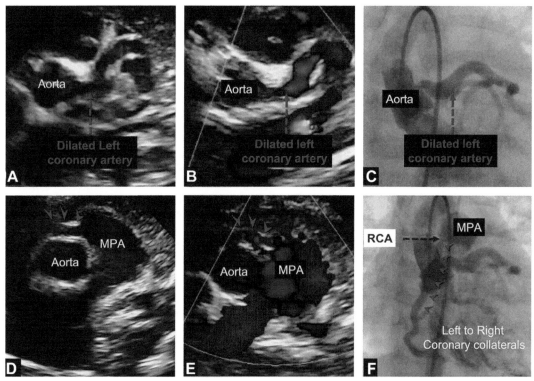

Fig. 10. ARCAPA in a healthy appearing 9-month-old infant who was referred for an evaluation of a heart murmur. Echocardiographic images demonstrated dilated left coronary artery with normal aortic origin and prograde flow (A–C), which then provides flow to the right coronary artery (RCA, *arrowheads*), which connects to the main pulmonary artery (MPA) with flow from RCA to MPA (D–F).

repair or translocation of the connection to the aortic root, if feasible.[130] Takeuchi described the procedure involving creation of a coronary tunnel inside the pulmonary artery to establish continuity between the aorta and the LCA ostium, in 1979.[131–133] This procedure was useful in cases in which direct implantation was thought to be difficult because of unfavorable coronary anatomy. Use of this method is declining given the high rate of complications including supravalvular pulmonary stenosis, intrapulmonary baffle leaks, and aortic valve insufficiency as well as a 30% chance of reoperation or catheter intervention over time. Thus, direct reimplantation has increasingly become the procedure of choice. Urgent corrective surgery to establish a two-coronary circulation is shown to lead to quick recovery of ventricular function in majority with excellent long-term survival.[131,134–137] A recent cohort study by Patel and colleagues described early surgical outcomes in 37 subjects with ALCAPA with short length of postoperative stay, low morbidity, and no surgical mortality. As in prior studies, they found more late complications with the Takeuchi procedure compared with direct reimplantation.[128] These patients had excellent status at

their long-term follow-up, with a significant improvement in the left ventricular ejection fraction and mitral valve regurgitation.[128,138,139] Despite normal ejection fraction, most patients had abnormal measurement of myocardial mechanics.[138]

Anomalous origin of the right coronary artery from the pulmonary artery

According to the latest American Heart Association/American College of Cardiology guidelines, repair is a Class I recommendation for symptomatic patients with ARCAPA and a Class IIa recommendation in asymptomatic patients with ventricular dysfunction or myocardial ischemia attributed to ARCAPA.[94] Surgical intervention consists of reimplantation of the RCA, including excising the anomalous origin of the RCA along with a button of the pulmonary arterial wall and translocating it into the anterior aspect of the ascending aorta.[114,130]

Recommendations to physical activities

Athletes with ALCAPA or ARCAPA can participate only in low-intensity class IA sports, whether or not they have had a prior myocardial infarction, and pending repair of the anomaly.[23] After repair of ALCAPA and ARCAPA, decisions regarding exercise restriction may be based on the presence of sequelae such as myocardial infarction or ventricular dysfunction.[23]

SUMMARY

Congenital coronary anomalies are not an infrequent occurrence, and their clinical presentation typically occurs during early years, although may be manifested only in adulthood. In the setting of AAOCA, this is particularly concerning because it inflicts sudden loss of healthy young lives. This event, although rare, leads to incalculable grief in families, organizations, and communities. An anomalous origin of one or more coronary arteries from the pulmonary artery is hemodynamically significant and produces myocardial ischemia leading to ischemic cardiomyopathy or SCD, thus surgical intervention in this setting is well defined. However, in AAOCA, current published consensus guidelines for the diagnosis and management of these abnormalities are limited by insufficient evidence due to lack of hard endpoints. There remains significant variability in risk stratification and management decisions, particularly in the asymptomatic patient. Standardized approach to the evaluation of these patients, with careful data collection and collaboration among centers, is likely the way to improve risk stratification and lead to optimal management decision. Such strategies will foster a safer environment for these patients to engage in exercise and sports participation, key components to successful and healthier lives.

CLINICS CARE POINTS

- Coronary artery anomalies may occur in up to 1% of the population and comprise the second most frequent cause of sudden death in the young.
- Echocardiography can diagnose up to 95% of patients, though advanced imaging is essential to define morphologic features.
- Myocardial functional studies under provocative stress are important in risk stratification.
- Surgical intervention may be indicated in a subset of patients.
- Exercise activities should be carefully considered as sedentarism is a great risk factor for lifetime cardiovascular disease.

DISCLOSURE

The authors have nothing to disclose.

REFERENCES

1. Angelini P, Velasco JA, Flamm S. Coronary anomalies: incidence, pathophysiology, and clinical relevance. Circulation 2002;105(20):2449–54.
2. Kayalar N, Burkhart HM, Dearani JA, et al. Congenital coronary anomalies and surgical treatment. Congenit Heart Dis 2009;4(4):239–51.
3. Maron BJ, Doerer JJ, Haas TS, et al. Sudden deaths in young competitive athletes analysis of 1866 deaths in the United States, 1980-2006. Circulation 2009;119(8):1085–92.
4. Angelini P. Coronary artery anomalies: an entity in search of an identity. Circulation 2007;115(10): 1296–305.
5. Basso C, Maron BJ, Corrado D, et al. Clinical profile of congenital coronary artery anomalies with origin from the wrong aortic sinus leading to sudden death in young competitive athletes. J Am Coll Cardiol 2000;35(6):1493–501.
6. Cheezum M, O'Gara P, Blankstein R, et al. Anomalous aortic origin of a coronary artery from the inappropriate sinus of Valsalva. J Am Coll Cardiol 2017; 69(12). https://doi.org/10.1016/j.jacc.2017.01.031.
7. Molossi S, Sachdeva S. Anomalous coronary arteries. Curr Opin Cardiol 2020;35(1):42–51.
8. Molossi S, Martínez-Bravo LE, Mery CM. Anomalous aortic origin of a coronary artery. Methodist Debakey Cardiovasc J 2017;15(2):111–21.
9. Mainwaring RD, Reddy VM, Reinhartz O, et al. Surgical repair of anomalous aortic origin of a coronary artery. Eur J Cardio-thoracic Surg 2014;46(1):20–6.
10. Sachdeva S, Frommelt MA, Mitchell ME, et al. Surgical unroofing of intramural anomalous aortic origin of a coronary artery in pediatric patients: single-center perspective. J Thorac Cardiovasc Surg 2018;155(4):1760–8.
11. Molossi S, Agrawal H. Clinical evaluation of anomalous aortic origin of a coronary artery (AAOCA). Congenit Heart Dis 2017;12(5):607–9.
12. Mainwaring RD, Murphy DJ, Rogers IS, et al. Surgical repair of 115 patients with anomalous aortic origin of a coronary artery from a single institution. World J Pediatr Congenit Hear Surg 2016;7(3): 353–9.
13. Frommelt PC, Berger S, Pelech AN, et al. Prospective identification of anomalous origin of left coronary artery from the right sinus of Valsalva using transthoracic echocardiography: importance of color Doppler flow mapping. Pediatr Cardiol 2001; 22(4):327–32.
14. Lorber R, Srivastava S, Wilder TJ, et al. Anomalous aortic origin of coronary arteries in the young

echocardiographic evaluation with surgical correlation. JACC Cardiovasc Imaging 2015;8(11): 1239–49.

15. de Jonge GJ, van Ooijen PMA, Piers LH, et al. Visualization of anomalous coronary arteries on dualsource computed tomography. Eur Radiol 2008; 18(11):2425–32.

16. Kacmaz F, Ozbulbul NI, Alyan O, et al. Imaging of coronary artery anomalies: the role of multidetector computed tomography. Coron Artery Dis 2008; 19(3):203–9.

17. Komatsu S, Sato Y, Ichikawa M, et al. Anomalous coronary arteries in adults detected by multislice computed tomography: presentation of cases from multicenter registry and review of the literature. Heart Vessels 2008;23(1):26–34.

18. Lee S, Uppu SC, Lytrivi ID, et al. Utility of multimodality imaging in the morphologic characterization of anomalous aortic origin of a coronary artery. World J Pediatr Congenit Heart Surg 2016;7(3):308–17.

19. Su JT, Chung T, Muthupillai R, et al. Usefulness of real-time navigator magnetic resonance imaging for evaluating coronary artery origins in pediatric patients. Am J Cardiol 2005;95(5):679–82.

20. Aljaroudi WA, Flamm SD, Saliba W, et al. Role of CMR imaging in risk stratification for sudden cardiac death. JACC Cardiovasc Imaging 2013;6(3): 392–406.

21. Brothers JA, Whitehead KK, Keller MS, et al. Cardiac MRI and CT: differentiation of normal ostium and intraseptal course from slitlike ostium and interarterial course in anomalous left coronary artery in children. AJR Am J Roentgenol 2015;204(1): W104–9.

22. Brothers JA, McBride MG, Seliem MA, et al. Evaluation of myocardial ischemia after surgical repair of anomalous aortic origin of a coronary artery in a series of pediatric patients. J Am Coll Cardiol 2007; 50(21):2078–82.

23. Van Hare GF, Ackerman MJ, Evangelista J-AK, et al. Eligibility and disqualification recommendations for competitive athletes with cardiovascular abnormalities: task force 4: congenital heart disease: a scientific statement from the American heart association and American College of Cardiology. Circulation 2015;132(22):e281–91.

24. Brothers JA, Frommelt MA, Jaquiss RDB, et al. Expert consensus guidelines: anomalous aortic origin of a coronary artery. J Thorac Cardiovasc Surg 2017;153(6):1440–57.

25. Doan TT, Bonilla-ramirez C, Sachdeva S, et al. Abstract 13007 : myocardial ischemia in anomalous aortic origin of a right coronary artery : medium-term follow-up in a large prospective cohort. Circulation 2020;142(suppl_3):A13007.

26. Qasim A, Doan TT, Pham TD, et al. Is exercise stress testing useful for risk stratification in anomalous aortic origin of a coronary artery? Semin Thorac Cardiovasc Surg 2022. In press.

27. Molossi S, Agrawal H, Mery CM, et al. Outcomes in anomalous aortic origin of a coronary artery following a prospective standardized approach. Circ Cardiovasc Interv 2020;13(2):e008445.

28. Mery CM, De León LE, Molossi S, et al. Outcomes of surgical intervention for anomalous aortic origin of a coronary artery: a large contemporary prospective cohort study. J Thorac Cardiovasc Surg 2018;155(1):305–19.e4.

29. Maeda K, Schnittger I, Murphy DJ, et al. Surgical unroofing of hemodynamically significant myocardial bridges in a pediatric population. J Thorac Cardiovasc Surg 2018;156(4):1618–26.

30. Cho S-H, Joo H-C, Yoo K-J, et al. Anomalous origin of right coronary artery from left coronary sinus: surgical management and clinical result. Thorac Cardiovasc Surg 2015;63(5):360–6.

31. Brothers J, Carter C, McBride M, et al. Anomalous left coronary artery origin from the opposite sinus of Valsalva: evidence of intermittent ischemia. J Thorac Cardiovasc Surg 2010;140(2):e27–9.

32. Paridon SM, Alpert BS, Boas SR, et al. Clinical stress testing in the pediatric age group: a statement from the American Heart Association council on cardiovascular disease in the young, committee on atherosclerosis, hypertension, and obesity in youth. Circulation 2006;113(15):1905–20.

33. Pellikka PA, Arruda-Olson A, Chaudhry FA, et al. Guidelines for performance, interpretation, and application of stress echocardiography in ischemic heart disease: from the American society of echocardiography. J Am Soc Echocardiogr 2020; 33(1):1–41. e8.

34. Chen MH, Abernathey E, Lunze F, et al. Utility of exercise stress echocardiography in pediatric cardiac transplant recipients: a single-center experience. J Hear Lung Transpl 2012;31(5):517–23.

35. El Assaad I, Gauvreau K, Rizwan R, et al. Value of exercise stress echocardiography in children with hypertrophic cardiomyopathy. J Am Soc Echocardiogr 2020;33(7):888–94.e2.

36. Badruddin SM, Ahmad A, Mickelson J, et al. Supine bicycle versus post-treadmill exercise echocardiography in the detection of myocardial ischemia: a randomized single-blind crossover trial. J Am Coll Cardiol 1999;33(6):1485–90.

37. Kimball TR. Pediatric stress echocardiography. Pediatr Cardiol 2002;23(3):347–57.

38. Armstrong WF, Zoghbi WA. Stress echocardiography: current methodology and clinical applications. J Am Coll Cardiol 2005;45(11):1739–47.

39. Thompson WR. Stress echocardiography in paediatrics: implications for the evaluation of anomalous aortic origin of the coronary arteries. Cardiol Young 2015;25(8):1524–30.

40. Pahl E, Duffy CE, Chaudhry FA. The role of stress echocardiography in children. Echocardiography 2000;17(5):507–12.

41. Ou P, Kutty S, Khraiche D, et al. Acquired coronary disease in children: the role of multimodality imaging. Pediatr Radiol 2013;43(4):444–53.

42. Deng ES, O'Brien SE, Fynn-Thompson F, et al. Recurrent sudden cardiac arrests in a child with an anomalous left coronary artery. JACC Case Rep 2021;3(13):1527–30.

43. Lameijer H, Kampman MAM, Oudijk MA, et al. Ischaemic heart disease during pregnancy or postpartum: systematic review and case series. Neth Hear J 2015;23(5):249–57.

44. Fabozzo A, DiOrio M, Newburger JW, et al. Anomalous aortic origin of coronary arteries: a single-center experience. Semin Thorac Cardiovasc Surg 2016;28(4):791–800.

45. Mumtaz MA, Lorber RE, Arruda J, et al. Surgery for anomalous aortic origin of the coronary artery. Ann Thorac Surg 2011;91(3):811–5.

46. Agati S, Secinaro A, Caldaroni F, et al. Perfusion study helps in the management of the intraseptal course of an anomalous coronary artery. World J Pediatr Congenit Hear Surg 2019; 10(3):360–3.

47. Blomjous MSH, Budde RPJ, Bekker MWA, et al. Clinical outcome of anomalous coronary artery with interarterial course in adults: single-center experience combined with a systematic review. Int J Cardiol 2021;335:32–9.

48. Doan TT, Molossi S, Sachdeva S, et al. Dobutamine stress cardiac MRI is safe and feasible in pediatric patients with anomalous aortic origin of a coronary artery (AAOCA). Int J Cardiol 2021;334:42–8.

49. Bonilla-Ramirez C, Molossi S, Sachdeva S, et al. Outcomes in anomalous aortic origin of a coronary artery after surgical reimplantation. J Thorac Cardiovasc Surg 2021;162(4):1191–9.

50. Hernandez-Pampaloni M, Allada V, Fishbein MC, et al. Myocardial perfusion and viability by positron emission tomography in infants and children with coronary abnormalities: correlation with echocardiography, coronary angiography, and histopathology. J Am Coll Cardiol 2003;41(4):618–26.

51. Greenwood JP, Maredia N, Younger JF, et al. Cardiovascular magnetic resonance and single-photon emission computed tomography for diagnosis of coronary heart disease (CE-MARC): a prospective trial. Lancet 2012;379(9814):453–60.

52. Schwitter J, Wacker CM, Wilke N, et al. MR-IMPACT II: magnetic Resonance Imaging for Myocardial Perfusion Assessment in Coronary artery disease Trial: perfusion-cardiac magnetic resonance vs. single-photon emission computed tomography for the detection of coronary artery disease: a comparative. Eur Heart J 2013;34(10):775–81.

53. Ge Y, Antiochos P, Steel K, et al. Prognostic value of stress CMR perfusion imaging in patients with reduced left ventricular function. JACC Cardiovasc Imaging 2020. https://doi.org/10.1016/j.jcmg.2020.05.034. Published online.

54. Wahl A, Paetsch I, Gollesch A, et al. Safety and feasibility of high-dose dobutamine-atropine stress cardiovascular magnetic resonance for diagnosis of myocardial ischaemia: experience in 1000 consecutive cases. Eur Heart J 2004;25(14):1230–6.

55. Paetsch I, Jahnke C, Wahl A, et al. Comparison of dobutamine stress magnetic resonance, adenosine stress magnetic resonance, and adenosine stress magnetic resonance perfusion. Circulation 2004;110(7):835–42. doi:.FB.

56. Jahnke C, Nagel E, Gebker R, et al. Prognostic value of cardiac magnetic resonance stress tests: adenosine stress perfusion and dobutamine stress wall motion imaging. Circulation 2007;115(13):1769–76.

57. Gebker R, Jahnke C, Manka R, et al. Additional value of myocardial perfusion imaging during dobutamine stress magnetic resonance for the assessment of coronary artery disease. Circ Cardiovasc Imaging 2008;1(2):122–30.

58. Charoenpanichkit C, Hundley WG. The 20 year evolution of dobutamine stress cardiovascular magnetic resonance. J Cardiovasc Magn Reson 2010;12(1):59.

59. Nagel E, Lehmkuhl HB, Bocksch W, et al. Noninvasive diagnosis of ischemia-induced wall motion abnormalities with the use of high-dose dobutamine stress MRI: comparison with dobutamine stress echocardiography. Circulation 1999;99(6):763–70.

60. Leong-Poi H, Rim S-J, Le DE, et al. Perfusion versus function: the ischemic cascade in demand ischemia: implications of single-vessel versus multivessel stenosis. Circulation 2002;105(8):987–92.

61. Hauser M, Bengel FM, Kühn A, et al. Myocardial blood flow and flow reserve after coronary reimplantation in patients after arterial switch and Ross operation. Circulation 2001;103(14):1875–80.

62. Hauser M, Kuehn A, Hess J. Myocardial perfusion in patients with transposition of the great arteries after arterial switch operation. Circulation 2003; 107(18):2001.

63. Secinaro A, Ntsinjana H, Tann O, et al. Cardiovascular magnetic resonance findings in repaired anomalous left coronary artery to pulmonary artery connection (ALCAPA). J Cardiovasc Magn Reson 2011;13(1):1–6.

64. Prakash A, Powell AJ, Krishnamurthy R, et al. Magnetic resonance imaging evaluation of myocardial perfusion and viability in congenital and acquired pediatric heart disease. Am J Cardiol 2004;93(5):657–61.

65. Noel C. Cardiac stress MRI evaluation of anomalous aortic origin of a coronary artery. Congenit Heart Dis 2017;12(5):627–9.

66. Pennell DJ, Sechtem UP, Higgins CB, et al. Clinical indications for cardiovascular magnetic resonance (CMR): consensus Panel report. Eur Heart J 2004; 25(21):1940–65.

67. Paetsch I, Jahnke C, Fleck E, et al. Current clinical applications of stress wall motion analysis with cardiac magnetic resonance imaging. Eur J Echocardiogr 2005;6(5):317–26.

68. Wilkinson JC, Doan TT, Loar RW, et al. Myocardial stress perfusion MRI using regadenoson: a weight-based approach in infants and young children. Radiol Cardiothorac Imaging 2019;1(4):e190061.

69. Doan TT, Wilkinson JC, Loar RW, et al. Regadenoson stress perfusion cardiac magnetic resonance imaging in children with Kawasaki disease and coronary artery disease. Am J Cardiol 2019;124(7): 1125–32.

70. Strigl S, Beroukhim R, Valente AM, et al. Feasibility of dobutamine stress cardiovascular magnetic resonance imaging in children. J Magn Reson Imaging 2009;29(2):313–9.

71. Scannell CM, Hasaneen H, Greil G, et al. Automated quantitative stress perfusion cardiac magnetic resonance in pediatric patients. Front Pediatr 2021;9:1–8.

72. Agrawal H, Wilkinson JC, Noel CV, et al. Impaired myocardial perfusion on stress CMR correlates with invasive FFR in children with coronary anomalies. J Invasive Cardiol 2021;33(1):E45–51. Available at: http://www.ncbi.nlm.nih.gov/pubmed/33385986.

73. Doan TT, Qureshi AM, Sachdeva S, et al. Beta-blockade in intraseptal anomalous coronary artery with reversible myocardial ischemia. World J Pediatr Congenit Hear Surg 2021;12(1):145–8.

74. Doan TT, Molossi S, Qureshi AM, et al. Intraseptal anomalous coronary artery with myocardial infarction: Novel surgical approach. Ann Thorac Surg 2020;110(4):e271–4.

75. Doan TT, Zea-Vera R, Agrawal H, et al. Myocardial ischemia in children with anomalous aortic origin of a coronary artery with intraseptal course. Circ Cardiovasc Interv 2020;13(3):e008375.

76. Agrawal H, Molossi S, Alam M, et al. Anomalous coronary arteries and myocardial bridges: risk stratification in children using Novel cardiac catheterization techniques. Pediatr Cardiol 2017;38(3): 624–30.

77. Bigler MR, Ashraf A, Seiler C, et al. Hemodynamic relevance of anomalous coronary arteries originating from the opposite sinus of Valsalva-in search of the evidence. Front Cardiovasc Med 2021;7. https://doi.org/10.3389/fcvm.2020.591326.

78. Doan TT, Wilkinson JC, Agrawal H, et al. Instantaneous wave-free ratio (iFR) correlates with fractional flow reserve (FFR) assessment of coronary artery stenoses and myocardial bridges in children. J Invasive Cardiol 2020;32(5):176–9. Available at: http://www.ncbi.nlm.nih.gov/pubmed/32357130.

79. Vatner SF, McRitchie RJ, Braunwald E. Effects of dobutamine on left ventricular performance, coronary dynamics, and distribution of cardiac output in conscious dogs. J Clin Invest 1974;53(5): 1265–73.

80. Asrress KN, Schuster A, Ali NF, et al. Myocardial haemodynamic responses to dobutamine stress compared to physiological exercise during cardiac magnetic resonance imaging. J Cardiovasc Magn Reson 2013;15(S1):15–6.

81. Bartunek J, Wijns W, Heyndrickx GR, et al. Effects of dobutamine on coronary stenosis physiology and morphology: comparison with intracoronary adenosine. Circulation 1999;100(3):243–9.

82. Escaned J, Cortés J, Flores A, et al. Importance of diastolic fractional flow reserve and dobutamine challenge in physiologic assessment of myocardial bridging. J Am Coll Cardiol 2003;42(2):226–33.

83. Sen S, Escaned J, Malik IS, et al. Development and Validation of a new adenosine-independent index of stenosis severity from coronary wave–intensity analysis. J Am Coll Cardiol 2012;59(15):1392–402.

84. Davies JE, Sen S, Dehbi H-M, et al. Use of the instantaneous wave-free ratio or fractional flow reserve in PCI. N Engl J Med 2017;376(19): 1824–34.

85. Petraco R, van de Hoef TP, Nijjer S, et al. Baseline instantaneous wave-free ratio as a pressure-only estimation of Underlying coronary flow reserve. Circ Cardiovasc Interv 2014;7(4):492–502.

86. Götberg M, Christiansen EH, Gudmundsdottir IJ, et al. Instantaneous wave-free ratio versus fractional flow reserve to guide PCI. N Engl J Med 2017;376(19):1813–23.

87. Doan TT, Qureshi AM, Gowda S, et al. Abstract 11876: instantaneous wave-free ratio and fractional flow reserve are helpful in the assessment of anomalous aortic origin of a coronary artery. Circulation 2021;144(Suppl_1):A11876Z.

88. Joanna G, Ann ML, Rukmini K, et al. Physiological evaluation of anomalous aortic origin of coronary arteries and myocardial bridges. J Am Coll Cardiol 2021;77(18_Supplement_1):514.

89. Aleksandric SB, Djordjevic-Đikic AD, Dobric MR, et al. Functional assessment of myocardial bridging with conventional and diastolic fractional flow reserve: vasodilator versus inotropic provocation. J Am Heart Assoc 2021;10(13). https://doi.org/10.1161/JAHA.120.020597.

90. Angelini P, Uribe C, Monge J, et al. Origin of the right coronary artery from the opposite sinus of Valsalva in adults: characterization by intravascular ultrasonography at baseline and after stent

angioplasty. Catheter Cardiovasc Interv 2015; 86(2):199–208.

91. Angelini P, Velasco JA, Ott D, et al. Anomalous coronary artery arising from the opposite sinus: descriptive features and pathophysiologic mechanisms, as documented by intravascular ultrasonography. J Invasive Cardiol 2003;15(9):507–14. Available at: http://www.ncbi.nlm.nih.gov/pubmed/12947211.

92. Driesen BW, Warmerdam EG, Sieswerda G-JT, et al. Anomalous coronary artery originating from the opposite sinus of Valsalva (ACAOS), fractional flow reserve- and intravascular ultrasound-guided management in adult patients. Catheter Cardiovasc Interv 2018;92(1):68–75.

93. Heyden CM, Brock JE, Ratnayaka K, et al. Intravascular ultrasound (IVUS) provides the filling for the angiogram's crust: benefits of IVUS in pediatric interventional Cardiology. J Invasive Cardiol 2021; 33(12):E978–85. Available at: http://www.ncbi.nlm.nih.gov/pubmed/34866050.

94. Stout KK, Daniels CJ, Aboulhosn JA, et al. 2018 AHA/ACC guideline for the management of adults with congenital heart disease: Executive summary: a report of the American College of Cardiology/American heart association task force on clinical practice guidelines. Circulation 2019;139(14):e637–97.

95. Brothers JA. Coronary artery anomalies in children: what is the risk? Curr Opin Pediatr 2016;28(5): 590–6.

96. Jacobs ML. Anomalous aortic origin of a coronary artery: the gaps and the guidelines. J Thorac Cardiovasc Surg 2017;153(6):1462–5.

97. Martínez-Bravo LE, Mery CM. Commentary: the intercoronary pillar—not necessarily an innocent bystander. J Thorac Cardiovasc Surg 2019; 158(1):218–9.

98. Mosca RS, Phoon CKL. Anomalous aortic origin of a coronary artery is not always a surgical disease. Semin Thorac Cardiovasc Surg Pediatr Card Surg Annu 2016;19(1):30–6.

99. Jegatheeswaran A, Devlin PJ, Williams WG, et al. Outcomes after anomalous aortic origin of a coronary artery repair: a Congenital Heart Surgeons' Society Study. J Thorac Cardiovasc Surg 2020; 160(3):757–71.e5.

100. Law T, Dunne B, Stamp N, et al. Surgical results and outcomes after reimplantation for the management of anomalous aortic origin of the right coronary artery. Ann Thorac Surg 2016;102(1):192–8.

101. Bonilla-Ramirez C, Molossi S, Caldarone CA, et al. Anomalous aortic origin of the coronary arteries – state of the art management and surgical techniques. Semin Thorac Cardiovasc Surg Pediatr Card Surg Annu 2021;24(Im):85–94.

102. Padalino MA, Franchetti N, Hazekamp M, et al. Surgery for anomalous aortic origin of coronary arteries: a multicentre study from the European Congenital Heart Surgeons Association. Eur J Cardio-thoracic Surg 2019;56(4):696–703.

103. Yerebakan C, Ozturk M, Mota L, et al. Complete unroofing of the intramural coronary artery for anomalous aortic origin of a coronary artery: the role of commissural resuspension? J Thorac Cardiovasc Surg 2019;158(1):208–17.e2.

104. Schubert SA, Kron IL. Surgical unroofing for anomalous aortic origin of coronary arteries. Oper Tech Thorac Cardiovasc Surg 2016;21(3):162–77.

105. Sharma V, Burkhart HM, Dearani JA, et al. Surgical unroofing of anomalous aortic origin of a coronary artery: a single-center experience. Ann Thorac Surg 2014;98(3):941–5.

106. Frommelt PC, Sheridan DC, Berger S, et al. Ten-year experience with surgical unroofing of anomalous aortic origin of a coronary artery from the opposite sinus with an interarterial course. J Thorac Cardiovasc Surg 2011;142(5): 1046–51.

107. Izumi K, Wilbring M, Stumpf J, et al. Direct reimplantation as an alternative approach for treatment of anomalous aortic origin of the right coronary artery. Ann Thorac Surg 2014;98(2):740–2.

108. Goda M, Meuris B, Meyns B. Right coronary translocation for anomalous origin of right coronary artery from the left coronary sinus. Interact Cardiovasc Thorac Surg 2011;13(2):201–2.

109. Jegatheeswaran A. Commentary: transection and reimplantation: Putting all your eggs in one basket? J Thorac Cardiovasc Surg 2021;162(4):1201–2.

110. Najm HK, Ahmad M. Transconal unroofing of anomalous left main coronary artery from right sinus with trans-septal course. Ann Thorac Surg 2019;108(6):e383–6.

111. Najm HK, Ahmad M, Hammoud MS, et al. Surgical Pearls of the transconal unroofing procedure - modifications and midterm outcomes. Ann Thorac Surg 2022. https://doi.org/10.1016/j.athoracsur.2022.04.027. Published online April 28.

112. Brotherton H, Philip RK. Anomalous left coronary artery from pulmonary artery (ALCAPA) in infants: a 5-year review in a defined birth cohort. Eur J Pediatr 2008;167(1):43–6.

113. Al-Dairy A, Rezaei Y, Pouraliakbar H, et al. Surgical repair for anomalous origin of the right coronary artery from the pulmonary artery. Korean Circ J 2017; 47(1):144–7.

114. Williams IA, Gersony WM, Hellenbrand WE. Anomalous right coronary artery arising from the pulmonary artery: a report of 7 cases and a review of the literature. Am Heart J 2006;152(5):1004.e9-17.

115. Rajbanshi BG, Burkhart HM, Schaff HV, et al. Surgical strategies for anomalous origin of coronary artery from pulmonary artery in adults. J Thorac Cardiovasc Surg 2014;148(1):220–4.

116. Doan TT, Khan A, Lantin-Hermoso MR. Is it Just a murmur? Part 1-3. 2019. Available at: https://www.acc.org/education-and-meetings/patient-case-quizzes/2019/09/12/13/29/is-it-just-a-murmur-part-1.

117. Bland EF, White PD, Garland J. Congenital anomalies of the coronary arteries: report of an unusual case associated with cardiac hypertrophy. Am Heart J 1933;8(6):787–801.

118. Wesselhoeft H, Fawcett JS, Johnson AL. Anomalous origin of the left coronary artery from the pulmonary trunk. Its clinical spectrum, pathology, and pathophysiology, based on a review of 140 cases with seven further cases. Circulation 1968;38(2):403–25.

119. Roberts WC, Robinowitz M. Anomalous origin of the left anterior descending coronary artery from the pulmonary trunk with origin of the right and left circumflex coronary arteries from the aorta. Am J Cardiol 1984;54(10):1381–3.

120. Roberts WC. Major anomalies of coronary arterial origin seen in adulthood. Am Heart J 1986;111(5):941–63.

121. Lerberg DB, Ogden JA, Zuberbuhler JR, et al. Anomalous origin of the right coronary artery from the pulmonary artery. Ann Thorac Surg 1979;27(1):87–94.

122. Kudumula V, Mehta C, Stumper O, et al. Twenty-year outcome of anomalous origin of left coronary artery from pulmonary artery: management of mitral regurgitation. Ann Thorac Surg 2014;97(3):938–44.

123. Birk E, Stamler A, Katz J, et al. Anomalous origin of the left coronary artery from the pulmonary artery: diagnosis and postoperative follow up. Isr Med Assoc J 2000;2(2):111–4. http://www.ncbi.nlm.nih.gov/pubmed/10804930.

124. Ojala T, Salminen J, Happonen J-M, et al. Excellent functional result in children after correction of anomalous origin of left coronary artery from the pulmonary artery–a population-based complete follow-up study. Interact Cardiovasc Thorac Surg 2010;10(1):70–5.

125. Kühn A, Kasnar-Samprec J, Schreiber C, et al. Anomalous origin of the right coronary artery from the pulmonary artery (ARCAPA). Int J Cardiol 2010;139(2):e27–8.

126. Winner MW, Raman SV, Sun BC, et al. Preoperative assessment of anomalous right coronary artery arising from the main pulmonary artery. Case Rep Med 2011;2011:642126.

127. Yu Y, Wang Q-S, Wang X-F, et al. Diagnostic value of echocardiography on detecting the various types of anomalous origin of the left coronary artery from the pulmonary artery. J Thorac Dis 2020;12(3):319–28.

128. Patel SG, Frommelt MA, Frommelt PC, et al. Echocardiographic diagnosis, surgical treatment, and outcomes of anomalous left coronary artery from the pulmonary artery. J Am Soc Echocardiogr 2017;30(9):896–903.

129. Hoffman JIE. Electrocardiogram of anomalous left coronary artery from the pulmonary artery in infants. Pediatr Cardiol 2013;34(3):489–91.

130. Kouchoukos NT, Blackstone EH, Hanley FL, et al. Chapter 46 - congenital anomalies of the coronary arteries. Kirklin/Barrat-Boyes Card Surg 2012;588–97. https://doi.org/10.1016/B978-0-7020-6929-1.00058-7.

131. Takeuchi S, Imamura H, Katsumoto K, et al. New surgical method for repair of anomalous left coronary artery from pulmonary artery. J Thorac Cardiovasc Surg 1979;78(1):7–11. Available at: http://www.ncbi.nlm.nih.gov/pubmed/449387.

132. Bunton R, Jonas RA, Lang P, et al. Anomalous origin of left coronary artery from pulmonary artery. Ligation versus establishment of a two coronary artery system. J Thorac Cardiovasc Surg 1987;93(1):103–8. Available at: http://www.ncbi.nlm.nih.gov/pubmed/3796022.

133. Isomatsu Y, Imai Y, Shin'oka T, et al. Surgical intervention for anomalous origin of the left coronary artery from the pulmonary artery: the Tokyo experience. J Thorac Cardiovasc Surg 2001;121(4):792–7.

134. Jin Z, Berger F, Uhlemann F, et al. Improvement in left ventricular dysfunction after aortic reimplantation in 11 consecutive paediatric patients with anomalous origin of the left coronary artery from the pulmonary artery. Early results of a serial echocardiographic follow-up. Eur Heart J 1994;15(8):1044–9.

135. Alexi-Meskishvili V, Hetzer R, Weng Y, et al. Anomalous origin of the left coronary artery from the pulmonary artery. Early results with direct aortic reimplantation. J Thorac Cardiovasc Surg 1994;108(2):354–62. Available at: http://www.ncbi.nlm.nih.gov/pubmed/8041183.

136. Cochrane AD, Coleman DM, Davis AM, et al. Excellent long-term functional outcome after an operation for anomalous left coronary artery from the pulmonary artery. J Thorac Cardiovasc Surg 1999;117(2):332–42.

137. Vouhé PR, Tamisier D, Sidi D, et al. Anomalous left coronary artery from the pulmonary artery: results of isolated aortic reimplantation. Ann Thorac Surg 1992;54(4):621–6. ; discussion 627.

138. Cabrera AG, Chen DW, Pignatelli RH, et al. Outcomes of anomalous left coronary artery from pulmonary artery repair: beyond normal function. Ann Thorac Surg 2015;99(4):1342–7.

139. Qasim A, Doan TT, Pham TDN, et al. Poster: exercise stress testing in risk stratification of anomalous aortic origin of a coronary artery. In: Pediatric Reseacrh Symposium at Texas Children's Hospital. 2021. Available at: https://www.texaschildrens.org/sites/default/files/uploads/documents/symposia/2021/posters/90.pdf 2021.

Cardiopulmonary Exercise Testing Interpretation in Athletes
What the Cardiologist Should Know

Mustafa Husaini, MD[a], Michael S. Emery, MD, MS[b],*

KEYWORDS

- Cardiopulmonary stress test • Rate of oxygen consumption(VO2) • Athlete

KEY POINTS

- Cardiopulmonary exercise testing (CPET) is used clinically for symptom assessment and quantification of functional capacity.
- Exercise physiology is different in competitive athletes and highly active persons (CAHAPs) compared to the general population.
- The choice of testing protocol and modality is imperative for proper interpretation of CPET results.
- Peak VO2, anaerboic threshold, chronotrophic index, oxygen pulse, SpO2, breathing reserve, and respiratory rate are different between CAHAPs and the general population.

Abbreviations	
CPET	Cardiopulmonary exercise testing
CAHAP	Competitive athlete and highly active person
VO2	Oxygen consumption
VCO2	Carbon dioxide production
VE	Minute ventilation
SV	Stroke volume
HR	Heart rate
a-vO2$_{diff}$	arteriovenous oxygen concentration difference

INTRODUCTION

Cardiopulmonary exercise testing (CPET), a valuable tool in medicine and sports performance for decades, couples traditional exercising testing parameters (electrocardiogram [ECG], blood pressure [BP], heart rate [HR], and peripheral oxygen saturation [SpO2]) with gas exchange measurement of oxygen consumption ($\dot{V}O2$) and carbon dioxide production ($\dot{V}CO2$) as well as ventilation ($\dot{V}E$). These later components allow for an integrated assessment of the cardiovascular, pulmonary, metabolic, and musculoskeletal systems. In clinical practice, CPETs are traditionally used for

[a] Department of Medicine, Division of Cardiovascular Medicine, Washington University School of Medicine, 4921 Parkview Place, Saint Louis, MO 63110, USA; [b] Sports Cardiology Center, Department of Cardiovascular Medicine, Heart, Vascular and Thoracic Institute, Cleveland Clinic Lerner College of Medicine of Case Western Reserve University, Cleveland Clinic, 9500 Euclid Avenue, Desk J2-4, Cleveland, OH 44195, USA
* Corresponding author. Department of Cardiovascular Medicine, Section of Clinical Cardiology, Heart, Vascular and Thoracic Institute, Cleveland Clinic, 9500 Euclid Avenue, Desk J2-4, Cleveland, OH 44195.
E-mail address: emerym2@ccf.org
Twitter: @husainim (M.H.); @MichaelEmeryMD (M.S.E.)

Cardiol Clin 41 (2023) 71–80
https://doi.org/10.1016/j.ccl.2022.08.006
0733-8651/23/© 2022 Elsevier Inc. All rights reserved.

unexplained dyspnea, exercise intolerance, stratification for heart or lung transplantation, and the quantification of functional capacity; serial comparisons incrementally improve diagnostic utility for a variety of cardiovascular conditions.[1]

There has been an increasing emphasis on evaluating cardiorespiratory fitness in clinical practice.[2] However, it is imperative that proper interpretation of CPET occurs and this is especially important when evaluating competitive athletes and highly active persons (CAHAPs). Exercise physiology in CAHAP has shown to be distinct compared with a nonathletic patient and/or the patient with overt cardio-pulmonary disease evaluated in most clinical laboratories; thus attention needs to be paid to the interpretation of CPET results in this unique population.[3]

DISCUSSION
Cardiopulmonary Exercise Test in Athletes

There are two key reasons a cardiologist would choose to perform a CPET in an athlete. The first is for medical testing that can aid in diagnosis by provoking symptoms during a true maximal stress test. The second reason is to improve performance as gas exchange parameters can pinpoint metabolic thresholds that aid in creating various exercise zones. Once a CPET is chosen as the appropriate testing modality, the next question becomes how to best perform the optimal test.

Traditional exercise testing has often used the Bruce Protocol that was described in 1950 by Dr Robert Bruce and has become ingrained into cardiac risk assessment, especially for coronary artery disease (CAD).[4–6] The standard Bruce protocol uses a treadmill at 1.7 miles per hour (MPH) at a 10° incline with an increase of approximately 2° and 1 mph every 3 min. Each successive stage increases the workload by approximately three metabolic equivalents; however, these large jumps in workload can obscure diagnostic precision.[7] The utilization of the Bruce protocol is rarely optimal in CAHAP as the goals of testing are different as is the underlying physiologic assumptions.[7–9] Many athletes can achieve high workloads, which results in steep inclines on the Bruce protocol. Two major issues with this high incline include (1) walking at a high grade does not reproduce the type of exercise most athletes perform and (2) many athletes are limited by calf discomfort related to the incline rather than cardiopulmonary exhaustion. Thus, it is imperative that the proper exercise protocol including modality be customized to the individuals' baseline fitness while allowing 8 to 12 min of exercise be used and interpreted within the appropriate clinical context.[10]

What are the determinants of human performance?

Three key components of human exercise performance are $\dot{V}O2$ max, lactate threshold, and work economy. The first two components can be readily assessed as part of a clinical CPET, whereas the latter often requires more complex protocols. For human skeletal muscles to function during normal exercise, the cardiovascular system must provide oxygenated blood to muscle mitochondria. By the Fick principle, $\dot{V}O2$ is equal to the cardiac output (CO) multiplied by the arteriovenous oxygen concentration difference (a-vO2$_{diff}$). The a-vO2$_{diff}$ is a function of how much oxygen is extracted at the cellular level whereas the CO is the stroke volume (SV) multiplied by the HR. Although central and peripheral adaptions occur with exercise training that contribute to increased exercise capacity, $\dot{V}O2$ max in healthy individuals at sea level is limited by the ability to deliver oxygen (CO) to exercising muscles regardless of training status rather than an inability to extract O2 in the periphery (a-vO2$_{diff}$).[11] Exercise-induced cardiac remodeling (EICR) is major determinate in the ability of an athlete to increase O2 delivery and increase $\dot{V}O2$ max, which has a strong correlation with the intensity, duration, and frequency of exercise with increased total volume correlating to more EICR.[12] During exercise, there will be a similar increase in heart rate but CAHAP with EICR will have much larger CO resulting from their increased SV manifesting as a larger $\dot{V}O2$ max.

What is the difference between peak $\dot{V}O2$ and true $\dot{V}O2$ max?

Historically, $\dot{V}O2$ max was established by performing multiple exercise stress tests. Each test would have a constant workload with subsequent tests having an incrementally greater workload until a true plateau in $\dot{V}O2$ could be shown despite the increasing workload hence establishing a $\dot{V}O2$ max (**Fig. 1**, left panel).[13] A $\dot{V}O2$ peak is the highest $\dot{V}O2$ that occurs without a plateau and is what is often seen in contemporary CPET evaluations with a single, continuously ramped workload work examination (see **Fig. 1**, right panel). It is uncommon to see a true $\dot{V}O2$max on a ramp protocol as there is not enough time within each stage to elicit a true plateau in $\dot{V}O2$. Because a plateau in $\dot{V}O2$ is rarely seen in single, incremental workload examination, we will be referring to $\dot{V}O2$ peak within this article as the highest $\dot{V}O2$ value obtained during a contemporary, single CPET.

True V̇O2 Max

"multiple tests with different work rates until true max elicited"

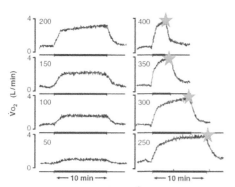

Peak V̇O2

"single test with increasing work; uncommon to see a true V̇O2 max"

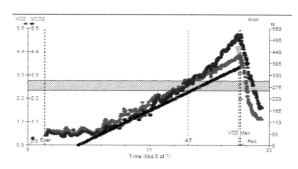

Fig. 1. Comparison of true V̇O2 max versus contemporary obtained peak V̇O2. Left panel: a true maximal V̇O2 (*green star*) can be obtained when multiple cardiopulmonary exercise tests are performed, each at a constant workload but increased relative to the previous test. Here, a true plateau in V̇O2 will be shown. Right panel: a peak V̇O2 (*orange triangle*) is often obtained in contemporary, single, continuously ramped workload CPET evaluations. *From:* Whipp and Mahler, Dynamics of pulmonary gas exchange during exercise: in west: Pulmonary Gas Exchange, Academic Press 1980.

Differences in Cardiopulmonary Exercise Test Parameters in Athletes Versus Nonathletes

Clinicians need to be aware of some fundamental differences in athletes that reflect normal physiology rather than a pathologic response as would be encountered in patients with heart and lung disease (**Table 1**).[14] Understanding the basics of exercise physiology in athletes can bring important perspectives to deciphering the meaning and significance of these parameters when deemed "abnormal". Complicating this interpretation is the fact that there is minimal normative data in athletes as traditional normative values have been derived in the general sedentary population, where there are expected differences in exercise physiology as compared with trained athletes. As such, commonly used V̇O2 max predication equations derived from general population cohorts perform poorly among competitive endurance athletes.[3] Furthermore, training-related adaptations may define CPET parameters, such as SpO2 and breathing reserve (BR), as abnormal despite no true pathology. It is thus imperative that cardiologists treating CAHAPs understand exercise physiology in athletes and its relationship to EICR when interpreting this information.

Cardiac output, stroke volume, and heart rate

At the start of exercise, the initial increase in CO is largely the result of increased venous return from skeletal muscle contraction and an increase in heart rate from removal of parasympathetic drive.[15,16] With continued exercise, the heart continues to appropriately augment CO with increased SV and coordination from the lungs to exchange carbon dioxide for oxygen and muscle mitochondria to produce energy from oxygen delivery. In healthy individuals and athletes, CO increases approximately 6 L for every 1 L increase in V̇O2.[17] Data suggest that the lower maximal HR in athletes emphasizes the role of enhanced SV as the driver of increased CO during exercise.[18] The cardiovascular system is typically the primary limiting factor in healthy individuals regardless of training status.[16] In athletes, there are four crucial cardiovascular CPET components that are important to consider differently compared with the untrained healthy individual: V̇O2 peak, O2 pulse, heart rate, and blood pressure.

V̇O2 peak As represented by the Fick principle, V̇O2 derives from the product of a-vO2$_{diff}$ and CO. In normal individuals (including elite-level athletes) at sea-level, the primary limiting factor to V̇O2max is CO. As maximum HR is determined by genetics, gender, and age, SV is the primary variable responsible for augmentation in V̇O2 max with training. Elite endurance athletes can generate remarkably high SVs by increasing end-diastolic volume owing to a compliant heart, distensible pericardium, and EICR.[19] Strength and mixed athletes may or may not have these physiologic adaptations and thus, can have V̇O2

Table 1
Various cardiopulmonary exercise testing parameters in athletes & nonathletes

CPET Parameter	Similar Between Athletes and Nonathletes	Can be Different in Some athletes
Metabolic/cardiovascular		
V̇O2		Peak V̇O2 can be significantly higher particularly with endurance athletes
AT		Occurs at a higher percentage of peak V̇O2 particularly with endurance athletes
Max HR	↔	Variable when using age predicted equations
CI		Often <0.8 owing to relative "normal" HR response with exceptional peak V̇O2 particularly in endurance athletes
V̇O2/h (O2 pulse)		Well above predicted values with potential plateau near peak exercise
RER	X	
V̇O2/work slope	X	
Ventilatory/gas exchange		
SpO2		EIAH can be seen near peak exercise in some athletes with very high peak V̇O2
PETCO2	X	
RC	X	
VE/V̇CO2 nadir/slope	↔	Slope can be elevated if taken through end exercise
Breathing reserve		Can be lower in athletes with exceptional fitness
RR		Can be higher (>50 breaths/min) in athletes usually with exceptional fitness

Abbreviations: AT, anaerobic threshold; CI, chronotropic index; EIAH, exercise-induced arterial hypoxemia; HR, heart rate; PETCO2, end-tidal carbon dioxide; RC, respiratory compensation; RER, respiratory exchange ratio; RR, respiratory reserve; SpO2, oxygen saturation; V̇CO2, rate of carbon dioxide production; V̇O2, rate of oxygen consumption.

max values in the "normal range" as predicted by age and gender matched controls.

Currently used reference standards are derived from the sedentary, general population and defines normal based on baseline demographics (eg, age, sex, race, and body mass), not their fitness. As such, the cardiologist should be aware of a possible normal V̇O2 max providing false reassurance in the symptomatic CAHAP with cardiac pathology. Clinical context, type/duration of prior training, and appropriate interpretation of other CPET parameters is thus imperative to ensure that cardiac pathology in physically fit patients is not missed.

Oxygen pulse O2 pulse is a mathematical construct derived by rearranging the Fick equation using measurements obtainable from a noninvasive CPET (V̇O2 and HR). Literally, this is the amount of oxygen consumed per heartbeat and is composed of the product of SV and a-vO2$_{diff}$:

$$O2\ Pulse = \frac{V\dot{O}2}{HR} = Stroke\ Volume\ X\ a$$
$$- vO2diff$$

$$O2\ Pulse = \frac{\dot{V}O2}{HR} = \frac{Stroke\ Volume}{a - vO2\ difference}$$

O2 pulse plateau below peak V̇O2 in a nonathlete

O2 pulse plateau near V̇O2 peak in an athlete

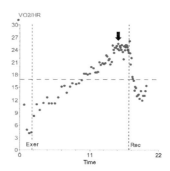

Fig. 2. Comparison of O2 pulse plateaus in athletes compared with nonathletes. Changes in stroke volume can be inferred from the trajectory of the O2 pulse during a graded workload cardiopulmonary exercise test. In nonathletes, the O2 pulse is often linear throughout exercise. Left panel: a plateau in the O2 pulse (*arrow*) within the general population can be a potential sign of myocardial ischemia. Right panel: athletes can have a plateau in their O2 pulse (*arrow*) and is likely a representation of a true V̇O2 max. *Horizontal line represents predicted peak O2 pulse.* Exer, onset of exercise; Rec, onset of recovery.

a-vO2$_{diff}$ is not generally a limiting factor at sea level in those without mitochondrial disease and increases linearly and predictably across the spectrum of exercise capacity.[20] As such, changes in SV can be inferred from the trajectory of the O2 pulse during a graded exercise effort.[21] However, it must be realized that the O2 pulse is not just SV, and it only infers the SV response to exercise and should not be used in an attempt to calculate true SV (ie, O2 pulse is NOT the amount of blood ejected from the left ventricle per beat).

Although SV normally plateaus during exercise in nonathletes and athletes at ~50% of V̇O2peak, O2 pulse tends be linear or curvilinear throughout exercise as it represents the product of a-vO2$_{diff}$ (which is linear throughout exercise) and SV. A commonly described pathologic feature in CPET is a plateau or decrease in O2 pulse with increasing work rates implying an impairment in SV during exercise and potential myocardial ischemia.[22] In the general population, clinical guidelines recommend that an O2 pulse plateau can be a useful addition to ECG testing for the detection of ischemic heart disease (**Fig. 2**, left panel).[22–24] In athletes, however, this phenomenon can be commonly seen despite having an O2 pulse peak well above predicted normal values and does not seem to correlate to obstructive CAD (see **Fig. 2**, right panel). In a study of elite soccer players, an O2 pulse plateau was seen in up to 20% during the last 2 min of testing.[25] In a separate a cohort of athletes who had CPET within 90 days of invasive or computed tomography

coronary angiography, an O2 pulse plateau was not a useful predictor for obstructive CAD.[26] Those with a plateau in their O2 pulse on CPET did not have obstructive CAD, were fitter and had a longer exercise ramp time. This phenomenon in athletes likely represents a true V̇O2max (rather than a V̇O2peak), a physiologic limitation of SV and/or oxygen extraction during intense exercise. Thus, it is imperative that the appropriate clinical context and other CPET parameters are used when interpreting an O2 pulse plateau.

Heart rate Heart rate increases linearly with exercise to increase CO although in some athletes a slight deflection to a lesser slope or a "breakpoint" heart rate can be seen corresponding to lactate threshold, referred to as the Conconi point.[16] The often-cited HR max = 220 – age equation, based on approximately 35 data points and no regression analysis,[27] can significantly over or underestimate the achieved HR in athletes and depends on the testing modality used.[18,28] Other equations have been proposed but are not as ubiquitously used in practice as the classic 220-age formula. The value of CPET testing is that the gas exchange parameters allow for a determination of a physiologic maximal effort indicating a true maximum HR was obtained and individualized to the athlete.

The chronotropic index (CI) is a comparison of the HR reserve to metabolic reserve at peak exercise and is essentially the slope in the relationship between HR to V̇O2 trajectory:

$$Chronotropic\ Index\ (CI) = \frac{\left(\frac{Peak\ HR\ -Baseline\ HR}{Predicted\ peak\ HR\ -Baseline\ HR}\right)}{\left(\frac{Peak\ V\dot{O}2\ -Baseline\ V\dot{O}2}{Predicted\ Peak\ V\dot{O}2\ -Baseline\ V\dot{O}2}\right)}$$

The interpretation of the CI depends on our understanding of the previously described differences in HR between athletes and the general population. The CI should be approximately 1.0 in those with a "normal" $\dot{V}O2$ peak with values < 0.8 considered chronotropic incompetence.[29,30] In athletes, it is not uncommon to see CI < 0.80 given the markedly higher $\dot{V}O2$ max (denominator of CI equation) and similar maximal HR (numerator of CI equation). Thus, CI < 0.80 in athletes with high $\dot{V}O2$ max is likely normal, driven by their higher $\dot{V}O2$ peak, and should not be labeled as chronotropic incompetence.

Blood pressure Hypertensive response to exercise has often been defined as a value exceeding the 90th percentile, equating to a systolic blood pressure (SBP) > 210 mm Hg in males and SBP > 190 mm Hg in females.[31] Healthy, asymptomatic individuals with normal resting blood pressure but hypertensive response on Bruce protocol treadmill tests is associated with significantly increased long-term risk of hypertension and major cardiovascular events.[32] In athletes that can push to very high workloads; however, blood pressure elevation is frequently seen, such as in a study of 2,419 normotensive adolescent, professional and master athletes where upper limits of maximal SBP were exceeded in 43% of men (SBP 204 ± 22 mm Hg [mean ± standard deviation]) and 28% of women (180 ± 17 mm Hg). The SBP response was more pronounced in endurance athletes and the DBP response was more pronounced in strength athletes.[33] The larger CO generated by athletes, compared with nonathletes, coupled with similar peripheral vascular responses is likely the etiology of this phenomenon. A study of 7,542 male Veterans, indexing peak SBP to external workload (metabolic equivalents of task [METS]) to obtain an SBP-MET slope was a better discriminator of the effect of exercise on the vasculature. In contrast to peak SBP, an SBP/MET slope above the median was associated with a 27% higher risk of mortality.[34] An elevation of blood pressure during exercise is not always considered pathologic particularly in those athletes achieving very high workloads.

Ventilation

In healthy individuals, lung capacity is not a limiting factor in exercise as the capacity of the pulmonary system during exercise often exceeds the demands required for gas exchange.[35] Despite this, many athletes have larger lung volumes than age matched controls likely representing genetic predisposition rather than a training adapation.[36]

Breathing reserve BR is a metric describing the percentage of maximal voluntary ventilation (MVV) that is not used during exercise with normal >15 to 20% at peak exercise:[22]

$$Breathing\ Reserve\ (BR) = \frac{\dot{V}E\ -\ MVV}{MVV} X\ 100$$

MVV can be directly measured during pretest spirometry or estimated as measured FEV1 X 35 to 40.[37] As many athletes have larger lung volumes compared with age matched controls, if MVV is underestimated in an athlete then BR can be reported as falsely low or even negative.[36] Even if correctly measured, some healthy athletes can show a similarly low BR indicating that the pulmonary capacity has been fully used. However, it often takes a highly motivated and exceptionally fit athlete with a $\dot{V}O2$ max well above predicted values for an athlete to show at BR of <10%. Caution should be made in labeling an athlete as having an abnormal pulmonary mechanical to exercise when their $\dot{V}O2$ peak is well above predicted values and are asymptomatic. Assessment of flow-volume loop mechanics and respiratory patterns during exercise could provide more insight in such cases particularly if an athlete reports subjective symptoms.

Ventilation/$\dot{V}CO2$ Over the course of exercise, minute $\dot{V}E$ increases in proportion to the metabolic rate to maintain arterial homeostasis.[38] VE is most tightly coupled to $\dot{V}CO2$ and the $\dot{V}E/\dot{V}CO2$ ratio is the "efficiency" of VE to remove CO2 during exercise. There are several methods to report $\dot{V}E/\dot{V}CO2$ with two of the most common being the slope throughout portions of exercise and the nadir during exercise. In much of the heart failure literature, the slope is taken to peak exercise that is used to include the "exaggerated" hyperventilatory drive that is a common manifestation of this pathology in the heart failure population. This method, with a threshold slope > 34, has been shown to have prognostic implications in this patient cohort.[39] The $\dot{V}E/\dot{V}CO2$ nadir is the lowest value during exercise and an established

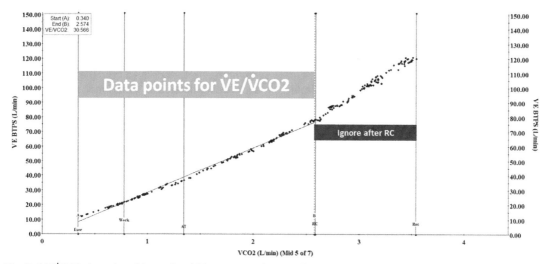

Fig. 3. VE/VCO2 slope in athletes should be measured up to the respiratory compensation point. Athletes often have a hyperventilatory drive after the respiration compensation point that increases the VE/VCO2 slope. In this population, the VE/VCO2 slope should be taken from the start of exercise to the respiratory compensation (RC) point.

alternative method with less variability than the slope method.[40]

In athletes, ventilatory efficiency seems fixed regardless of athletic training status.[41] It is not unusual, however, to observe VE/VCO2 values above normal particularly when the slope is taken to peak exercise. As athletes often have a pronounced hyperventilatory drive after the respiratory compensation (RC) point, the VE/VCO2 slope through end-exercise is not reflective of true ventilatory inefficiency in those capable of exercising well above their RC. In this situation, the elevated slope observed above RC can falsely imply impaired ventilatory efficiency despite no evidence of pathology. Thus, in athletes the VE/VCO2 should be calculated as the slope up to RC or by the VE/VCO2 nadir (**Fig. 3**).

Metabolism and gas exchange

Lactate homeostasis and the anaerobic threshold Through the process of cellular respiration, there are several metabolic thresholds that occur, which have clinical relevance. Before oxidative metabolism becomes completely "ramped up" during exercise, initial energy is derived from phosphocreatine (less than 10 s) and anaerobic metabolism (up to around 90 s).[42] In this initial portion of exercise, the production of lactate remains near resting levels as it is cleared at equal rates to production. After the first few minutes of exercise, oxidative metabolism becomes the primary source of energy. As exercise proceeds and the muscle metabolic needs are not met by oxidative metabolism, anaerobic metabolism increases with a corresponding increase in

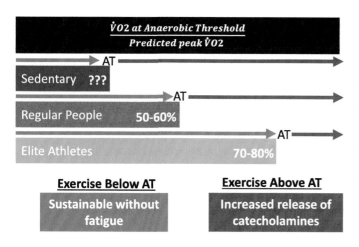

Fig. 4. Ratio of VO2 at anaerobic threshold to maximum VO2 differs by fitness level. The ratio of VO2 at the anaerobic threshold (AT) to the predicted peak VO2 is a useful marker for the evaluation of fitness. Exercise below AT is sustainable without cardiorespiratory fatigue. Elite endurance athletes reach AT at a higher VO2 (absolute level and relative to their predicted peak VO2) which explains their capacity to exercise with less cardiorespiratory fatigue at similar workloads compared with nonathletes.

lactate production. This increased production exceeds the body's clearance mechanisms with a subsequent increase in blood lactate. This is buffered by the bicarbonate buffering system resulting in additional CO2 being produced, which drives an increase in VE. Here, the $\dot{V}CO2$ is increased relative to $\dot{V}O2$ and can be defined on CPET through the steepening of the slope between these two parameters.[43] The physiologic phenomenon is often referred to as the anaerobic threshold (AT), the laboratory change as the lactate threshold, and the CPET determination as the first ventilatory threshold.[44]

Exercise below the AT is sustainable without cardiorespiratory fatigue while exercise after the threshold, where lactate production exceeds clearance, is not. Consistent endurance exercise creates cardiovascular and musculoskeletal adaptions that prolong the time of primary aerobic oxidative metabolism before anaerobic metabolism is required to generate further energy expenditure.[45,46] A metric to quantify this is the $\dot{V}O2$ at AT relative to the maximum $\dot{V}O2$ with higher percentages seen in more endurance-trained athletes. A normal ratio is 45% to 65% with endurance athletes having higher ratios, approaching 80% to 90%.[16] The general population and patients with cardiovascular disease have a much lower ratio that implies that AT occurs early in the course of oxidative metabolism, thus explaining the fatiguing physical activity that occurs with low levels of exertion (**Fig. 4**).

Exercise-induced arterial hypoxemia In endurance athletes with very high $\dot{V}O2$ max (eg, > 60–70 mL/kg/min or 150%–200% predicted), approximately ~50% will have an absolute reduction in arterial oxygen saturation (SaO2) ≤95% (or 3% <rest) during exercise at or near sea level with desaturations ranging from 3% to 15% from resting values.[47,48] This occurs at or near maximal exertion and does not seem to imply clinical pathology in the absence of symptoms or structural heart disease. EIAH is often not seen in true clinical practice as athletes are rarely pushed to this level of physical exertion and the fidelity of the typical finger pulse-oximeter is not high enough to reliably capture these desaturations. As such, the clinician needs to verify a high-quality waveform before reporting "abnormal" values or ascribing any potential clinical implications.

SUMMARY

CPET in CAHAP is an important test that can be used for diagnosis (provoking symptoms during a truly maximal test), potential risk stratification

and performance (metabolic thresholds to define training zones). Differences in physiology and exercise-induced cardiac remodeling could result in certain CPET parameters, when compared with normal values derived from the general population, being defined as "abnormal" despite no evidence of cardiovascular or pulmonary pathology. Understanding the uniqueness of exercise physiology in athletes can establish important perspectives in deciphering the meaning and significance of these parameters, as well as the metabolic relationships that can aid in creating training programs.

CLINICS CARE POINTS

- Cardiopulmonary exercise testing (CPET) can provide insight for both diagnosis and performance.
- Traditional exercise testing and interpretation in competitive athletes and highly active persons (CAHAPs) is often inadequate for proper clinical management of this unique population.
- There are numerous differences in CPET parameters in athletes that reflect normal physiology rather than a pathologic response to exercise.
- The $\dot{V}O2$ at anaerobic threshold to the predicted $\dot{V}O2$ is a useful metric to quantify fitness and helps explain the fatiguing physical activity that occurs in nonathletes, compared with athletes, at low levels of exertion.

DISCLOSURE

M. Husaini—none; M.S. Emery—none.

REFERENCES

1. Chaudhry S, Arena R, Bhatt DL, et al. A practical clinical approach to utilize cardiopulmonary exercise testing in the evaluation and management of coronary artery disease: a primer for cardiologists. Curr Opin Cardiol 2018;33(2):168–77.

2. Ross R, Blair SN, Arena R, et al. Importance of assessing cardiorespiratory fitness in clinical practice: a case for fitness as a clinical vital sign: a scientific statement from the American heart association. Circulation 2016;134(24):e653–99.

3. Petek BJ, Tso JV, Churchill TW, et al. Normative cardiopulmonary exercise data for endurance athletes: the

cardiopulmonary health and endurance exercise registry (CHEER). Eur J Prev Cardiol 2021;29(3):536–44.

4. Bruce RA, Blackmon JR, Jones JW, et al. Exercising testing in adult normal subjects and cardiac patients. Pediatrics 1963;32:SUPPL 742–756.

5. Shaw LJ, Peterson ED, Shaw LK, et al. Use of a prognostic treadmill score in identifying diagnostic coronary disease subgroups. Circulation 1998; 98(16):1622–30.

6. Mark DB, Hlatky MA, Harrell FE, et al. Exercise treadmill score for predicting prognosis in coronary artery disease. Ann Intern Med 1987;106(6):793–800.

7. Sarma S, Levine BD. Beyond the Bruce protocol: advanced exercise testing for the sports cardiologist. Cardiol Clin 2016;34(4):603–8.

8. Churchill TW, Disanto M, Singh TK, et al. Diagnostic yield of customized exercise provocation following routine testing. Am J Cardiol 2019;123(12):2044–50.

9. Sirico F, Fernando F, Di Paolo F, et al. Exercise stress test in apparently healthy individuals - where to place the finish line? The Ferrari corporate wellness programme experience. Eur J Prev Cardiol 2019; 26(7):731–8.

10. Gibbons RJ, Balady GJ, Bricker JT, et al. ACC/AHA 2002 guideline update for exercise testing: summary article. A report of the American college of cardiology/American heart association task force on practice guidelines (committee to update the 1997 exercise testing guidelines). J Am Coll Cardiol 2002;40(8):1531–40.

11. Bassett DR, Howley ET. Limiting factors for maximum oxygen uptake and determinants of endurance performance. Med Sci Sports Exerc 2000;32(1):70–84.

12. Baggish AL, Battle RW, Beckerman JG, et al. Sports cardiology: core curriculum for providing cardiovascular care to competitive athletes and highly active people. J Am Coll Cardiol 2017;70(15):1902–18.

13. Whipp BJ, Mahler M. Dynamics of pulmonary gas exchange during exercise, West J.B. In: *Pulmonary Gas Exchange* vol. II.. New York: Academic Press; 1980.

14. Emery M. Cardiopulmonary exercise testing in athletes: pearls and pitfalls. In. ACC.org Expert Analysis. 2021.

15. Saito M, Tsukanaka A, Yanagihara D, et al. Muscle sympathetic nerve responses to graded leg cycling. J Appl Physiol (1985) 1993;75(2):663–7.

16. Sarma S, Levine BD. Exercise physiology for the clinicianPaul D, Thompson ABF, editors. Exercise and Sports Cardiology. Europe: World Scientific; 2018. p. 23–62.

17. Hermansen L, Ekblom B, Saltin B. Cardiac output during submaximal and maximal treadmill and bicycle exercise. J Appl Physiol 1970;29(1):82–6.

18. Whyte GP, George K, Shave R, et al. Training induced changes in maximum heart rate. Int J Sports Med 2008;29(2):129–33.

19. Levine BD. VO2max: what do we know, and what do we still need to know? J Physiol 2008;586(1):25–34.

20. Stringer WW, Hansen JE, Wasserman K. Cardiac output estimated noninvasively from oxygen uptake during exercise. J Appl Physiol (1985) 1997;82(3):908–12.

21. Crisafulli A, Piras F, Chiappori P, et al. Estimating stroke volume from oxygen pulse during exercise. Physiol Meas 2007;28(10):1201–12.

22. Balady GJ, Arena R, Sietsema K, et al. Clinician's Guide to cardiopulmonary exercise testing in adults: a scientific statement from the American Heart Association. Circulation 2010;122(2):191–225.

23. Mezzani A, Agostoni P, Cohen-Solal A, et al. Standards for the use of cardiopulmonary exercise testing for the functional evaluation of cardiac patients: a report from the Exercise Physiology Section of the European Association for Cardiovascular Prevention and Rehabilitation. Eur J Cardiovasc Prev Rehabil 2009;16(3):249–67.

24. VAN DE Sande DAJP, Schoots T, Hoogsteen J, et al. O2 pulse patterns in male master athletes with normal and abnormal exercise tests. Med Sci Sports Exerc 2019;51(1):12–8.

25. Perim RR, Signorelli GR, Myers J, et al. The slope of the oxygen pulse curve does not depend on the maximal heart rate in elite soccer players. Clinics (Sao Paulo). 2011;66(5):829–35.

26. Petek BJ, Churchill TW, Sawalla Guseh J, et al. Utility of the oxygen pulse in the diagnosis of obstructive coronary artery disease in physically fit patients. Physiol Rep 2021;9(21):e15105.

27. RA R, Landwehr R. The surprising history of the "HRmax=220-age" equation. Int J Online Eng 2002;5:1–10.

28. Faff D, Ladyga M, Klusiewicz A, et al. Maximal heart rate in athletes. Biol Sport 2007;24:129–42.

29. Brubaker PH, Kitzman DW. Chronotropic incompetence: causes, consequences, and management. Circulation 2011;123(9):1010–20.

30. Gulati M, Shaw LJ, Thisted RA, et al. Heart rate response to exercise stress testing in asymptomatic women: the st. James women take heart project. Circulation 2010;122(2):130–7.

31. Schultz MG, Otahal P, Cleland VJ, et al. Exercise-induced hypertension, cardiovascular events, and mortality in patients undergoing exercise stress testing: a systematic review and meta-analysis. Am J Hypertens 2013;26(3):357–66.

32. Allison TG, Cordeiro MA, Miller TD, et al. Prognostic significance of exercise-induced systemic hypertension in healthy subjects. Am J Cardiol 1999;83(3):371–5.

33. Pressler A, Jähnig A, Halle M, et al. Blood pressure response to maximal dynamic exercise testing in an athletic population. J Hypertens 2018;36(9):1803–9.

34. Hedman K, Cauwenberghs N, Christle JW, et al. Workload-indexed blood pressure response is superior to

peak systolic blood pressure in predicting all-cause mortality. Eur J Prev Cardiol 2020;27(9):978–87.

35. McKenzie DC. Respiratory physiology: adaptations to high-level exercise. Br J Sports Med 2012;46(6): 381–4.

36. Dempsey JA, La Gerche A, Hull JH. Is the healthy respiratory system built just right, overbuilt, or underbuilt to meet the demands imposed by exercise? J Appl Physiol (1985) 2020;129(6):1235–56.

37. Society AT, Physicians ACoC. ATS/ACCP Statement on cardiopulmonary exercise testing. Am J Respir Crit Care Med 2003;167(2):211–77.

38. Collins S, Phillips DB, Brotto AR, et al. Ventilatory efficiency in athletes, asthma and obesity. Eur Respir Rev 2021;30(161).

39. Gitt AK, Wasserman K, Kilkowski C, et al. Exercise anaerobic threshold and ventilatory efficiency identify heart failure patients for high risk of early death. Circulation 2002;106(24):3079–84.

40. Sun XG, Hansen JE, Garatachea N, et al. Ventilatory efficiency during exercise in healthy subjects. Am J Respir Crit Care Med 2002;166(11):1443–8.

41. Salazar-Martínez E, de Matos TR, Arrans P, et al. Ventilatory efficiency response is unaffected by fitness level, ergometer type, age or body mass index in male athletes. Biol Sport 2018;35(4):393–8.

42. Gastin PB. Energy system interaction and relative contribution during maximal exercise. Sports Med 2001;31(10):725–41.

43. Beaver WL, Wasserman K, Whipp BJ. A new method for detecting anaerobic threshold by gas exchange. J Appl Physiol (1985) 1986;60(6):2020–7.

44. Poole D, Rossiter H, Brooks G, et al. The anaerobic threshold: 50+ years of controversy. J Physiol 2021; 599:737–67.

45. Jamnick NA, Pettitt RW, Granata C, et al. An examination and critique of current methods to determine exercise intensity. Sports Med 2020;50(10):1729–56.

46. Faude O, Kindermann W, Meyer T. Lactate threshold concepts: how valid are they? Sports Med 2009; 39(6):469–90.

47. Dempsey JA, Wagner PD. Exercise-induced arterial hypoxemia. J Appl Physiol (1985) 1999;87(6): 1997–2006.

48. Constantini K, Tanner DA, Gavin TP, et al. Prevalence of exercise-induced arterial hypoxemia in distance runners at sea level. Med Sci Sports Exerc 2017;49(5):948–54.

Devices and Athletics
Decision-Making Around Return to Play

Bradley Kay, MD, Rachel Lampert, MD*

KEYWORDS

- Implantable cardioverter defibrillator • athlete • sports • exercise

KEY POINTS

- Athletes with implantable cardiac defibrillators (ICDs) are a heterogenous group, including underlying disease process and specific indications for the devices.
- In the largest studies to date of athletes participating in sports with an ICD, while athletes did receive both appropriate and inappropriate shocks, these were not more frequent during sports participation than other activity, and there were no sports-related deaths or need for external resuscitation in the 440 athlete cohort (median followup 44 months.)
- While historically an ICD was considered an absolute contraindication to participation in sports beyond minimal intensity, guidelines now emphasize a shared decision-making approach for these athletes.
- Higher rate-cutoffs and longer arrhythmia detection thresholds have been associated with fewer shocks, without an increase in adverse events. There has been no association to date with outcomes in terms of number of leads or intravenous versus subcutaneous system, although the latter is largely understudied in athletes.

BACKGROUND

Sudden cardiac arrest (SCA) is an important cause of morbidity and mortality in young people, estimated to occur in up to 1 in 23,000 athletes.[1] All cases of SCA in the young are tragic; the high visibility of those occurring during sports participation can create a sense of tragedy throughout a community. Etiologies of SCA in the young include channelopathies, cardiomyopathies, congenital coronary anomalies or other congenital cardiac conditions.[1]

Defined by the Bethesda Conferences, an athlete is one who participates in an organized team or individual sport that requires regular competition against others as a central component, places a high premium on excellence and achievement, and requires some form of systematic (and usually intense) training.[2] Overall prevalence of SCA varies by study, but one of the largest prospective studies found the overall incidence in an adolescent and young adult cohort to be about 1 in 100,000 patient-years, with up to 2.3 in 100,000 in athletes.[3] A study of National Collegiate Athletic Association athletes found a similar incidence that was greatest in male basketball players—8.8 per 100,000 patient-years. This study also found an increase in SCA rates in higher divisions of competition (Division I) compared with lower divisions (Division II and III),[1] which may suggest a correlation with the intensity of training/competition and SCA.

Survival from SCA remains dismally low; less than 6% of patients with out of hospital cardiac arrest survive to discharge[4] and thus the prevention of SCA is critical. This can include an implantable cardioverter defibrillator (ICD) for those identified as at risk, through symptoms, such as syncope

The authors have nothing to disclose.
Section of Cardiovascular Medicine, Yale School of Medicine, 789 Howard Avenue, Dana 319, New Haven, CT 06520, USA
* Corresponding author.
E-mail address: rachel.lampert@yale.edu

Cardiol Clin 41 (2023) 81–92
https://doi.org/10.1016/j.ccl.2022.08.007
0733-8651/23/© 2022 Elsevier Inc. All rights reserved.

or resuscitated arrhythmia, preparticipation screening, or family screening.[5,6]

Once an athlete receives an ICD, many wish to continue competition. Until recently, based on the guidance of the 2005 Bethesda Conference, which offered a simple binary—yes/no—approach to sports participation, recommendation was for restriction for nearly all sports, except low intensity—class 1A sports.[2] In the absence of data at the time, concerns of the writing committee included the potential inability of the device to convert an arrhythmia at high-intensity exercise, and fear of injury due to arrhythmia or shock. Concern for system damage, particularly in pacemaker-dependent athletes, led to recommendations against participation in sports that potentially involve bodily trauma. For pacemaker patients, particularly those who are pacemaker-dependent, concerns regarding lead malfunction have led to restrictions from contact sports.

Weighing into the decision about sports participation is also the pitfalls of nonparticipation, not just on cardiovascular health, but on psychological well-being. For athletes, overall mental health is improved in those who are able to participate.[7] Inability to participate in sports for many adolescents has been the most difficult part of receiving an ICD.[8] For many athletes, sports participation is a way of life, and inherent in their decisions about playing are calculated risks.

SAFETY OF SPORTS FOR PATIENTS WITH IMPLANTABLE CARDIOVERTER DEFIBRILLATORS

The 2005 Bethesda Conference was largely based on expert consensus with few supporting data. To address this paucity of data, as a first step, surveys were sent to physician members of Heart Rhythm Society (HRS), inquiring about patients with an ICD who still opted to participate in vigorous exercise/sports, with greater than 40% reporting at least one such patient, and no adverse events were noted.[9] While surveys are prone to biases, these preliminary data prompted the creation of the ICD Sports Safety Registry to track these patients and monitor for events.

In 2013, the first results from this registry were published,[10] with the full cohort and full follow-up described in 2017.[11] The investigators looked at the primary composite endpoint of a serious adverse event during or within 2 hours of activity defined as (1) tachyarrhythmic death/externally resuscitated tachyarrhythmia or (2) severe injury requiring hospitalization resulting from a shock or syncopal episode and secondary endpoints of (1) appropriate and inappropriate shocks, (2)

multiple shocks within 1 appropriate shock episode, (3) moderate injury, requiring emergency room visit associated with shock, and (4) ICD lead/system damage including definite lead malfunction. The most frequent diagnosis was Long QT Syndrome (LQTS), followed by hypertrophic cardiomyopathy (HCM) and arrhythmogenic right ventricular cardiomyopathy (ARVC); 3% of the cohort had ICDs for a primary cardiac indication of catecholaminergic polymorphic ventricular tachycardia (CPVT) About half of athletes had an ICD placed for secondary prevention. The most common sports were running, basketball, and soccer.

None of the 440 patients in the final cohort met the primary end point at a median follow-up of 44 months (IQR 30–48 months). There were two deaths in the cohort, which were not related to physical activity. Twenty-eight percent of the cohort received a total of 184 shocks, 36% of which were during competition or practice and 30% of which occurred at rest. Ten percent received appropriate shocks (for VT/VF) during competition or practice, a rate of 3 per 100 person-years (**Table 1**). Shocks of any kind were more common during practice/competition compared with rest (20% vs 10%, $P<.0001$), but there was no difference in numbers of individuals receiving shocks during competition/practice compared with other physical activity (12% vs 10%, $P = .56$). Episodes requiring multiple shocks had a rate of 0.5 per 100 person-years, and were not significantly associated with activity (either competition/practice or other physical activity) compared with rest.

Quality of life was not assessed in the ICD Sports Registry. However, while some athletes stopped sports after receiving a shock, most returned, implying that the negative impact of shock on quality of life, was outweighed by the benefits to the quality they perceived from sports.

Lead failure is one of the feared complications of sports participation with devices. In a subanalysis of the ICD Sports Registry, Link and colleagues and found that 8% of patients had a lead malfunction; 4% of patients received inappropriate shocks due to this. Overall, the lead survival free of malfunction was 95% at 5 years and 89% at 10 years, similar to that in unselected cohorts.[12] There was an association of lead malfunction with age less than 21 at device implant, as well as leads under recall [Medtronic Fidelis (HR: 4.09) and Abbott Riata leads (HR: 3.13)]. Device type and access site did not predict malfunction. The only sport-related factors were yearly weightlifting hours in the highest tertile (greater than 104 hours, HR: 3.1). Contrary to the prior

Table 1
Number of shock events and of individuals receiving shocks

Rhythm	Competition Related, n[a]	Physical Activity Related, n[b]	Rest, n	Total, n (%)
Total cohort				
VT	29/21	15/11	19/13	63/41 (9)
VF	12/10	9/8	14/9	35/25 (6)
VT/VF storm	4/4	3/3	2/2	9/9 (2)
NSVT	1/1	0	0	1/1 (1)
SR	8/7	4/3	1/1	13/10 (2)
AF	7/5	14/10	4/4	25/14 (3)
Other SVT	3/3	4/4	1/1	8/8 (2)
SR strom	0	1/1	0	1/1 (1)
AF/SVT storm	0	2/2	0	2/2 (1)
T-wave oversensing	2/2	3/2	3/3	8/7 (2)
Noise	1/1	7/7	11/10	19/17 (4)
Total	67/51	62/46	55/42	184/121 (28)
Highly competitive subgroup				
VT	1/1	5/5	2/2	8/3 (3)
VF	4/3	3/1	5/2	12/4 (4)
VT/VF storm	1/1	0	0	1/1 (1)
AF	1/1	2/1	0	3/2 (2)
Other SVT	0/0	2/2	2/2	4/4 (5)
AF/SVT storm	0/0	1/1	0/0	1/1 (1)
T-wave oversensing	1/1	2/1	2/2	5/4 (5)
Noise	1/1	1/1	1/1	3/3 (3)
Total	9/8	16/13	12/8	37/25

Values refer to the number of events/number of unique individuals. Percents refers to percent of study population.

Among the total cohort, 33 shocks did not have available implantable cardioverter-defibrilator-stored data; the diagnosis is based on that of the treating physician. Of these, 12 were ventricular arrhythmia, 4 SVT, 13 noise, and 3 other. Among the highly competitive subgroup, 6 shocks did not have available implantable cardioverter-defibrilator-stored data; 3 noise, 1 VF, 1 T-wave oversensing, and 1 other SVT.

Abbreviations: AF, atrial fibrillation; NSVT, nonsustained ventricular tachycardia; SR, sinus rhythm; SVT, supraventricular; VF, ventricular fibrillation; VT, ventricular tachycardia.

[a] Includes competition, postcompetition, or practice for competition.
[b] Includes physical activity and postphysical activity.

From Lampert R, Olshansky B, Heidbuchel H, Lawless C, Saarel E, Ackerman M, Calkins H, Estes NAM, Link MS, Maron BJ, Marcus F, Scheinman M, Wilkoff BL, Zipes DP, Berul CI, Cheng A, Jordaens L, Law I, Loomis M, Willems R, Barth C, Broos K, Brandt C, Dziura J, Li F, Simone L, Vandenberghe K, Cannom D. Safety of Sports for Athletes With Implantable Cardioverter-Defibrillators: Long-Term Results of a Prospective Multinational Registry. Circulation. 2017 Jun 6;135(23):2310-2312.

belief, participation in sports with the heaviest use of arms or contact sports was not associated with lead malfunction, although numbers were small and these effects cannot be excluded.[13] (**Table 2**) There were no generator malfunctions in the registry.[11]

FACTORS IMPACTING RISK
Sports-Related Considerations

Risks to the patient or system may vary with specific sports. For example, in sports such as downhill skiing, swimming, or rock climbing whereby an athlete's survival relies on their ability to continue physically functioning, the risk of a sudden loss of control needs to be considered. In the ICD Sports Registry, injury was not seen in athletes participating in "high-risk" sports, but numbers were few. Analogously, motor vehicle accidents have not been shown to increase in patients with ICDs.

The risk of system damage in contact sports is another important factor to discuss with the

Table 2
Baseline characteristics: lead malfunction (exact test was used unless otherwise specified)

Variable	Unadjusted Hazard Ratio (95% CI)	P Value
Age at implant, y; and number of individuals in the age group		.42
10–19; n = 111	3.0 (0.8–11.3)	
20–29; n = 84	2.9 (0.8–10.8)	
30–39; 77	1.9 (0.5–8.1)	
40–49; n = 84	1.7 (0.4–7.2)	
50–60; n = 84	1.00	
Age <21 vs ≥21	2.19 (1.07–4.49)	.03
Age at enrollment, y	0.75 (0.58–0.98)/10y	.04
Sex (female vs male)	1.5 (0.7–3.1)	.26
Ejection fraction	1.03 (0.995–1.075)	.08
LVEF %≤50	3.2 (0.8–13.9)	.11
ICD indication (primary or secondary)	0.7 (0.3–1.5)	.35
Structural heart disease	1.5 (0.7–3.0)	.27
Contact		.69
Full contact vs limited	1.4 (0.6–3.1)	
Full contact vs noncontact	1.3 (0.5–3.4)	
Limited vs noncontact	1.0 (0.4–2.4)	
Use of arm		.46
Medium vs none	0.8 (0.4–1.7)	
Medium vs major	3.0 (0.4–22.7)	
None vs major	3.6 (0.5–27.7)	
Venous implant site (subclavian/axillary vs cephalic)	1.1 (0.5–2.7)	.78
Number of leads		.25
1 vs 2	0.5 (0.3–1.1)	
1 vs 3	0.8 (0.1–5.8)	
2 vs 3	1.4 (0.2–10.6)	
Lead family		.0027
Fidelis vs other	4.09 (1.82–9.17)	.0006
Fidelis vs Rieta	1.31 (0.47–3.60)	.61
Rieta vs others	3.13 (1.20–8.33)	.02
Lifetime weight listing; highest tertile vs others	0.7 (0.1–3.1)	.59
Yearly weight listing; highest tertile vs others	3.1 (1.1–8.9)	.04
History of prior lead malfunction	0.98 (0.34–2.81)	.97
History of prior lead extraction	0.87 (0.26–2.86)	.82

Abbreviations: ICD, implantable cardioverter defibrilator; LVEF, left ventricular ejection fraction.
From Link MS, Sullivan RM, Olshansky B, Cannom D, Berul CI, Hauser RG, Heidbuchel H, Jordaens L, Krahn AD, Morgan J, Patton KK, Saarel EV, Wilkoff BL, Li F, Dziura J, Brandt C, Barth C, Lampert R. Implantable Cardioverter Defibrillator Lead Survival in Athletic Patients. Circ Arrhythm Electrophysiol. 2021 Mar;14(3):e009344.

athlete when addressing return to play. While the ICD Sports Registry included many athletes participating in soccer and basketball, considered by the American Academy of Pediatrics to be contact sports, there were few athletes participating in intense contact sports such as hockey or football. System damage, regardless of the type of system (transvenous or subcutaneous) can lead to missensing and inappropriate/undelivered shocks or failure of pacing. At present, the data do not support the significant risk of system damage with any specific sport, but due to low overall numbers in the studies performed, the data remain unclear.[13]

Table 3
Athletes who participated in competitive college sports

Athlete	Cardiac Diagnosis	ICD Indication	Sex	Sport
1	LQTS	Prophylactic	F	Volleyball
2	LQTS	Syncope	M	Baseball
3	Dilated CM	Positive EPS	M	Paintball league
4	LQTS	VF/arrest	F	Soccer
5	LQTS	Syncope	F	Lacrosse
6	LQTS	Syncope	F	Triathlons
7	ARVC	Prophylactic	M	Soccer
8	LQTS	Syncope	F	Soccer
9	HCM	VF/arrest	M	Basketball
10	Congenital (TOF)	Syncope	M	Baseball
11	LQTS	Prophylactic	F	Soccer[a]
12	LV noncompaction	VF/arrest	M	Baseball
13	LQTS	Syncope	F	Tennis
14	Brugada	Syncope/positive EPS	M	Track and Field Cross country running
15	Idiopathic VT/VF (normal heart)	VF/arrest	M	Baseball
16	CPVT	VF/arrest	F	Tennis
17	LQTS	Prophylactic	M	Cross country running
18	Other	VF/arrest	M	Basketball[a]
19	LQTS	Prophylactic	M	Baseball[a]
20	LQTS	VF/arrest	F	Tennis

Abbreviations: ARVC, arrhythmogenic right ventricular cardiomyopathy; CM, cardiomyopathy; CPVT, catecholaminergic polymorphic ventricular tachycardia; EPS, electrophysiology study; F, female; HCM, hypertrophic cardiomyopathy; ICD, implantable cardioverter-defibrillator; LQTS, long QT syndrome; LV, left ventricular; M, male; TOF, tetralogy of Fallot; VF, ventricular fibrillation; VT, ventricular tachycardia.
[a] Division 1.
From Saarel EV, Law I, Berul CI, Ackerman MJ, Kanter RJ, Sanatani S, Cohen MI, Berger S, Fischbach PS, Burton DA, Dziura J, Brandt C, Simone L, Li F, Olshansky B, Cannom DS, Lampert RJ. Safety of Sports for Young Patients With Implantable Cardioverter-Defibrillators: Long-Term Results of the Multinational ICD Sports Registry. Circ Arrhythm Electrophysiol. 2018 Nov;11(11):e006305.

Also, some medications, such as beta blockers and diuretics may be completely or partially banned depending on the governing body of the sport. This may affect an athlete's ability to adhere to their ideal medication regimen if they wish to continue participation in competitive sports.[14]

Sports Intensity

To what extent the level of intensity of the sport influences the likelihood of arrhythmia, remains unclear. In the primary study, the most highly competitive, those participating in interscholastic sports, were not more likely to receive shocks during competition or practice, than those competing at lower levels[11] (**Table 3** for details of collegiate athletes).[15] However, while only competitive athletes were enrolled in the US, European sites also included "auto-competitive" recreational athletes—defined as those engaging in intense physical activity at least twice weekly (2 hours) with the aim to improve their physical performance limits but without competitive participation. In comparison, these recreational athletes were found to have fewer ICD shocks (13.8% vs 26.5%) during physical activity, due to fewer inappropriate shocks (2.5% vs 12%) when compared with the competitive cohort. Further, there was no difference in cessation of sports between competitive or recreational groups nor differences in the rates of lead malfunction. Whether there is a degree of intensity at which rates of ICD shocks may be greater in competitive athletes is not determined. Overall, outcomes in competitive and recreational athletic cohorts appear similar.[16]

Disease State

In discussion with an athlete considering returning to play, consideration of the underlying disease is critical. While the ICD terminated all ventricular arrhythmias in the ICD Sports Registry, notably, the only clinical variable associated with appropriate shocks during competition in the ICD Sports Registry, was the presence of ARVC, and these patients, were the most likely to receive multiple shocks during exercise. Further, while the ICD Sports Registry did not evaluate whether sports participation impacted the progression of underlying disease, prior studies have shown that for individuals with desmosomal mutations, exercise is associated with more arrhythmia complications, greater heart failure burden, and progression to meeting clinical criteria for ARVC in a dose-dependent manner.[17] One study from 2015, investigating ARVC outcomes based on athlete status found higher risk of ventricular tachyarrhythmia or death in competitive athletes, compared with either recreational athletes or inactive subjects; however, there was no difference for this outcome for recreational athletes, even those practicing high-dynamic sports, versus inactive subjects.[18]

Several factors are associated with arrhythmia in hypertrophic cardiomyopathy (HCM), including increased gradients across LVOT, degree of hypertrophy, and exercise-induced NSVT[19] and guidelines favor ICD placement. In the ICD Sports Registry, these patients, the second most-frequent diagnosis, were less likely to receive shocks during sports activity than those with other diagnoses, and none received multiple shocks during exercise.[10,11,16] Whether exercise impacts the progression of disease is unknown. In a mouse model of HCM, exercise prevented fibrosis, myocyte disarray, and induction of "hypertrophic" markers when initiated before established HCM pathology. Also, when initiated in older animals with established HCM pathology, exercise reversed myocyte disarray (but not fibrosis) and "hypertrophic" marker induction.[20] Human data are lacking on the long-term effects of extensive vigorous exercise in HCM.[19]

Long QT syndrome (LQTS) is commonly identified in those with SCA. The LQTS cohort in the ICD Sports Registry study represented about one-fifth of the total registry participants and none of these athletes had events requiring greater than one shock to terminate. One disease-specific study[21] found a very low rate of events in athletes with LQTS—one ICD shock in 650 athlete years—though it should be noted that that study only had 20 patients with ICDs, and notably about half were genotype-positive/phenotype-negative which may suggest an inherently lower-risk cohort.

There are few data on the safety of sports for patients with catecholaminergic polymorphic ventricular tachycardia (CPVT), with or without an ICD. Of the twelve athletes in the ICD Sports Registry with CPVT, one suffered multiple shocks during exercise.[10,11] It has been long suggested that subjects with CPVT should not receive an ICD due to the risk of exacerbation of electrical storm. However, while the increases in catecholamines with exercise may seem intuitively unsafe for these patients, one analysis of athletes with CPVT, all of whom were receiving appropriate treatment, found that, although athletes had more cardiac events before their diagnosis of CPVT when compared with non-athletes, there was no difference between events at follow-up, including ICD shocks.[22] Further, there is evidence that exercise in CPVT mutated mice may actually decrease arrhythmia burden,[23] and a small human study showed an increase in the threshold for the development of ventricular arrhythmia after a 12-week exercise program, compared with sedentary controls.[24]

Idiopathic VT/VF (iVF) has been felt to carry lower risk of recurrent arrhythmia. Three of the 48 athletes with this diagnosis in the ICD Registry, had multiple shocks from physical activity.[10,11,16] It is possible these may represent missed diagnoses of CPVT, and thus missed opportunity for appropriate treatment.

Coronary artery disease (CAD), represented in about one-tenth of the total subjects of the ICD Sports Registry, surprisingly, was the most common diagnosis associated with multiple shocks, in 3/45 athletes.[10,11,16] As asymptomatic atherosclerotic disease is a common cause of SCA in athletes,[25] stress testing, as well as aggressive risk reduction, and potentially more aggressive revascularization has been recommended.[26]

Prior Events

It has previously been well-established that a strong risk for ventricular arrhythmias and thus shocks is a prior history of shocks, with rates ranging from 10% to greater than 50% within 1 year in some studies,[27–30] regardless of physical activity status; newer programming methods and medications have decreased this burden. Although there was no statistical difference in the registry studies presented above between primary and secondary prevention ICDs,[10,11,16] the possibility of recurrent arrhythmia and potential shock needs to be discussed.

CURRENT GUIDELINES

Both American[5,6,19,31,32] and the European[33,34] statements and guidelines have provided recommendations regarding return to play for athletes with defibrillators. Current recommendations from all involved professional societies have made important changes from prior documents.[35] While nuanced differences exist, all have moved away from the prior binary recommendations toward the more nuanced class of recommendation approach. The current US AHA/ACC eligibility recommendations now consider competitive sports for an ICD patient IIB, "may be considered" while the ESC describes that shared decision-making should be considered as a IIA recommendation, "should be considered." The AHA/ACC eligibility document does not use the wording, "shared decision making," but an element of SDM is inherent in the IIB recommendation. For patients with HCM, the most common cardiomyopathy in athletes, recent AHA guidelines also specifically recommend shared-decision-making around return to play for athletes, with or without an ICD, although the prior eligibility statement continues to consider HCM a disqualifying condition.

The European guidelines emphasize the importance of considering all factors related to a patient's participation, including what they refer to as the "4 D's" of danger (to themselves or others by losing bodily control during sport), disease, device (pacemaker vs ICD, number of leads, device settings, shielding of generator) and dysrhythmia. The consensus statements emphasize shared decision-making once all factors previously mentioned are addressed and an overlying theme in the management of any athlete is the optimization of treatment of the underlying process. There is further specificity in the European documents around factors to take into consideration; for some, the restriction remains recommended related to the underlying condition, such as QT cutoffs in the long QT syndrome, or specific risk-markers in HCM, moderate-severe hypertrophy, history of SCA, LVOT obstruction greater than 50 mm Hg or blood pressure drop more than 25 mm Hg.[5,6,32,33] As many of these characteristics would in the US be considered an indication for an ICD, data from the ICD Sports Registry would then support their decision to continue sports if desired.

All statements and guidelines agree that an ICD should not be placed for the purpose of sports participation, in the absence of other indications for an ICD. For most disease entities, it is unknown to what degree athletic participation increases risk in a patient who has undergone standard evaluation which has not revealed high risk. ICD implantation is not without risk, and there can be long-term adverse events such as inappropriate shocks, or lead malfunction, which are acceptable if the device is otherwise indicated as potentially lifesaving, but not minimal.

SHARED DECISION MAKING
Return to Play

Shared decision-making is the most important part of the patient–doctor relationship. Like informed consent, shared decision-making ensures that the patient understands the risks and benefits of proposed options, in this case, return to play in sports. In studies of decision-making around medical treatment options, several studies have demonstrated greater patient satisfaction and fewer undecided patients, as well as better quality of life when shared decision-making is used.[36–38] This stands in contrast to the previously oft-employed paternalistic approach, whereby the doctor informs the patient what the course of treatment would be.

Decision-making around return to play is complex, and many athletes, even those eventually allowed to return, report a chaotic and frustrating process. In a mixed-methods interview study of 30 athletes with recent diagnoses of arrhythmogenic cardiac disease, the athletes had seen a median of 2 physicians and up to 7 physicians, with more than half of the athletes were disqualified from further competition by their first cardiologist. Six had to meet with administrators with 4 asked to sign waivers and 3 hired lawyers to contest disqualifications. These culminated in 2 athletes changing schools and 2 losing scholarships.[39] Athletes expressed frustration with poor communication, perceived lack of physician knowledge of their diagnosis, and unilateral, paternalistic decision-making, as well as cynicism that physicians and schools were primarily concerned with liability. This speaks to the immensely complex and daunting endeavor that the return to play experience can become for athletes. Shared decision-making is crucial for the well-being of the athlete.

There is no set script for a shared decision-making conversation pertaining to return to play. The discussion should start with the available data, including the limitations of that data and areas of uncertainty. How closely the athlete's own clinical situation, including their disease entity and sport, is reflected in the study population and how these may influence risk, as described above, should be discussed. Open-ended questions about the athlete's own values follow, with the issues that need to be considered as the athlete is considering return, such as the possibility of shocks. In most cases, data do not exist to allow the citation of specific risks. However, physicians can explain concepts of risk-tolerance that may help athletes and families put this decision in context.

Many of these conversations will not just be had with the athletes, but also with their parents and loved ones. It is important to help facilitate the discussion, but the physician should not serve as an intermediary for disputes among athletes and their parents.

Not Returning to Play

Decision for the cessation of athletic competition may be made, whether due to significant unavoidable risk of morbidity or mortality or if a shock is received and negative psychological outcomes result. As previously stated, this decision should not be made in a paternalistic fashion and rather through discussion with the athlete and their loved ones. It should be noted that athletes who are no longer participating in sports are not immune to arrhythmias and shocks; these patients may fill their time with other activities which may then trigger arrhythmias, such as video games, which have been reported to cause ventricular arrhythmias and SCA in susceptible individuals,[40] as well as the fact that in certain situations, such as CPVT, less exercise is associated with lower threshold for arrhythmia.[23,24] Some level of physical activity should be encouraged in almost any situation.

MANAGEMENT AFTER THE DECISION TO RETURN TO PLAY

Once an athlete has made the decision to return, optimizing disease-specific therapies (and making sure that the athlete has means of acquiring prescribed medications and understands their importance), optimizing device settings, and optimizing surroundings through ensuring an adequate emergency action plan (EAP) is crucial for safe return to play. For athletes with conditions exacerbated by extreme heat, such as Brugada Syndrome, LQTS, and CPVT, avoidance of peak sun hours in the summer and frequent water breaks can save lives and avoid trauma. Avoidance of exacerbating medications, dehydration, and electrolyte abnormalities is critical.[33] Communication amongst all stakeholders is also key after an athlete returns to play. Schools, coaches, and trainers should be involved in the return to play process and informed of the EAP, so as to act quickly in case of an event.

Disease-Specific Measures

Generally, for athletes with coronary artery disease minimizing ischemic burden is associated with decreased arrhythmic events and death.[41] Although not specifically studied in athletes, evaluating for and treating ischemia stands as a reasonable intervention before beginning activity and at intervals during long-term follow-up.

Left sympathetic denervation surgery has been suggested to reduce arrhythmia burden in both CPVT and LQTS in nonathlete populations.[42] Efficacy in decreasing arrhythmia specifically in response to sports participation has not been studied, but this intervention may also play a role. AHA recommends that athletes with monomorphic VT amenable to catheter ablation should undergo catheter ablation and restrict activity for at least 3 months and those undergoing suppressive therapy with medications wait at least 3 months after the last VT episode, before return.[6]

Device Programming and Monitoring

Device settings are a critical component of the management of athletes with devices. For pacemakers, ideal settings revolve around appropriate rate response strategies for age, allowing the patient's heart rate to increase appropriately while active. ICD programming is directed toward treating life-threatening ventricular arrhythmias and avoiding syncope while also avoiding inappropriate shocks for supraventricular tachyarrhythmias or sinus tachycardia.

In the general ICD population, higher rate cutoffs compared with conventional programming have been associated with decreased mortality and decreased rates of both appropriate and inappropriate therapies.[43,44]

A subanalysis of the ICD registry analyzing very high (heart rate >240 bpm), high (≥200 bpm) and low-rate (<200 bpm) cutoffs published in 2019 similarly found fewer total and inappropriate shocks with higher rate cutoffs, 15% versus 32% for appropriate shocks and 2% versus 9% for inappropriate shocks. Long duration alone— defined as greater than nominal as compared with "out-of-the-box"—was not associated with fewer total shocks; however, those with both high threshold and longer duration were found to have the fewest total and competition/practice-related shocks. There was no increase in syncope seen in those with higher cut-offs/longer durations. No difference was found between single- and dual-chamber ICDs in shock frequency.[45] **(Fig. 1)** These data suggest that, when appropriate, a combination of high threshold and longer

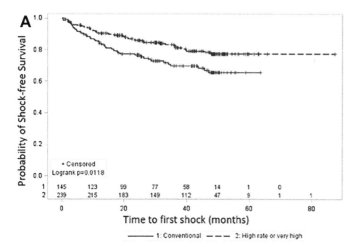

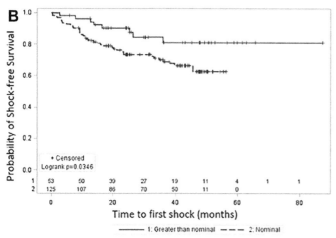

Fig. 1. Freedom from shock (including appropriate and inappropriate exclusive of noise/T-wave oversensing). (*A*): Rate cutoff: conventional versus high or very high rate. (*B*): Duration: nominal versus greater than nominal. (*From* Olshansky B, Atteya, G, Cannom, D, et al. Competitive athletes with implantable cardioverter–defibrillators—How to program? Data from the Implantable Cardioverter–Defibrillator Sports Registry. Heart Rhythm. 2019;16(4):581-587.)

detection duration can be beneficial in lowering shock burden. Specific patient factors can affect the ideal arrhythmia detection parameters and thus settings need to be personalized.

Although remote monitoring/interrogation data were not obtained in the registry, standard of care, based on expert consensus from the Heart Rhythm Society of remote monitoring of ICDs every 3 to 6 months should be used and pacemakers every 6 to 12 months as several meta-analyses have shown a reduction in costs and improved mortality with remote monitoring.[46] Current wireless monitoring systems can identify lead malfunction early.

Choice of Device

The ideal device for an athlete remains undetermined. First implanted in 2010, and approved by the Food and Drug Administration in 2012,

subcutaneous ICDs (S-ICD) have been shown to provide equal protection from SCA. Whether they will be preferable for athletes has not yet been investigated, as the ICD Sports Safety Registry included only patients with transvenous devices; data on S-ICDs in athletes are limited to case reports. Theoretically, lead malfunction may be less common with the S-ICD, in avoiding the "subclavian crush syndrome" due to friction between the clavicle and first rib. While the ICD Sports Registry did not show that sports with repetitive arm/shoulder motions such as rowing, increased the risk of damage to the leads, numbers may have been insufficient. The initial study of these systems in 2010 and then later the PRAETORIAN Investigators demonstrated noninferiority when compared with transvenous systems in terms of successful defibrillation and arrhythmia detection in nonathlete cohorts.[47] S-ICD systems are often preferred as the device type in young children, due to anatomic restrictions with the device through the venous system as well as longer-term risks of severe tricuspid regurgitation or infection. A registry of athletes with S-ICDs is expected to be starting shortly.

A newer minimally invasive, epicardial ICD has recently been studied primarily in children, involving a thoracotomy and intraabdominal location of the generator. Potential advantages of this technique are that the generator is more protected from damage due to trauma, as well as the fact that these devices can pace, unlike their S-ICD counterparts.[48] Similar to S-ICD though, there is a paucity of data on athletes, and longevity of this type of system is not described.

Emergency Action Plan

Emergency action plans (EAPs) are crucial for a safe return to play. While our interview study revealed that nearly 90% of the athletes had an emergency action plan on returning to play, in half the cases, this had been left to the athlete and family.[39] These should be in place for all sports organizations and venues; the presence of a player with an ICD should prompt a review. The emergency action plan should include a nearby automated external defibrillator (AED), and basic life support-capable coaches and teammates, in case the system is damaged and cannot deliver life-saving therapies. AEDs should be checked on a regular basis. Bystander CPR is well documented to improve outcomes in cardiac arrest. Using magnets in the event of inappropriate shocks is controversial and the authors recommend against that in the absence of a provider trained in their use as whether shocks are appropriate may not be apparent. Communications systems need to be in place with integration with local emergency medical services.[49]

SUMMARY

In the past decade, significant strides have been made in investigating the safety of athletic participation for patients with intracardiac devices. Previously felt to be a contraindication for participation, newer data from prospective registries suggest that the risks are likely lower than initially believed. A shared decision-making approach is critical for sports participation for those with intracardiac devices. Further research is needed in the realm of device choice, and on long-term effects of vigorous and/or competitive exercise for some underlying conditions, but overall, sports participation carries a low risk for many athletes with intracardiac devices.

DISCLOSURES

Dr Lampert has disclosures–in the past year, has received advisory board reimbursements, honoraria, and research support from Medtronic, and honoraria and research support from Abbott.

CLINICS CARE POINTS

- Shared decision-making ensuring is the most important aspect of the decision to return to play with an ICD. Ensuring the athlete is aware of the data and potential risks associated with returning to play, while helping athletes and families consider their own risk-tolerance and the role of competitive sports in their lives, is critical.

- Further interventions to reduce likelihood of shocks – either appropriate or inappropriate – should be discussed prior to return to play, including ablation or left sympathetic denervation in appropriate patients. The gaps in knowledge about applicability to athletes specifically should also be addressed, in order to set appropriate expectations.

- Optimization of medications and defibrillator programming is key to preventing ICD discharges, both appropriate and inappropriate.

- Emergency action plans are mandatory for all athletes returning to play with an ICD in place, where athletes, trainers and coaches are all aware of the plan in the event of emergency.

ACKNOWLEDGMENTS

The ICD Sports Registry received funding from Medtronic, Boston Scientific, and Abbott/St Jude.

REFERENCES

1. Harmon KG, Asif IM, Klossner D, et al. Incidence of sudden cardiac death in National collegiate athletic association athletes. Circulation 2011;123:1594–600.
2. Myerburg R, Estes NAM III, Fontaine JM, et al. 36th Bethesda conference: eligibility recommendations for competitive athletes with cardiovascular abnormalities - task force 10: automated external defibrillators. J Am Coll Cardiol 2005;45(8):1369–71.
3. Corrado D, Basso C, Rizzoli G, et al. Does sports activity enhance the risk of sudden death in adolescents and young adults? J Am Coll Cardiol 2003; 42(11):1959–63.

4. 2015 IoM. Strategies to improve cardiac arrest survival: a time to act. Washington, DC: The National Academies Press; 2015.

5. Maron B, Udelson JE, Bonow RO, et al. Eligibility and disqualification recommendations for competitive athletes with cardiovascular abnormalities: task force 3: hypertrophic cardiomyopathy, arrhythmogenic right ventricular cardiomyopathy and other cardiomyopathies, and myocarditis. Circulation 2015;132(22):e273–80.

6. Zipes D, Link MS, Ackerman MJ, et al. Eligibility and disqualification recommendations for competitive athletes with cardiovascular abnormalities: task force 9: arrhythmia and conduction defects: a scientific statement from the American heart association and American College of cardiology. Circulation 2015;132:e315–25.

7. McAllister D, Motamedi AR, Hame SL, et al. Quality of life assessment in elite collegiate athletes. Am J Sports Med 2001;29(6):806–10.

8. Rahman B, Macciocca I, Sahhar M, et al. Adolescents with implantable cardioverter defibrillators: a patient and parent Perspective. Pacing Clin Electrophysiol 2012;35:62–72.

9. Lampert R, Cannom D, Olshansky B. Safety of sports participation in patients with implantable cardioverter defibrillators: a survey of herat rhythm society members. J Cardiovasc Electrophysiol 2006;17(1):11–5.

10. Lampert R, Olshansky B, Heidbuchel H, et al. Safety of sports for athletes with implantable cardioverter-defibrillators: results of a prospective, multinational registry. Circulation 2013;127:2021–30.

11. Lampert R, Olshansky B, Heidbuchel H, et al. Safety of sports for athletes with implantable cardioverter-defbrillators: long-term results of a prospective multinational registry. Circulation 2017;135(23):2310–2.

12. Providencia R, Kramer DB, Pimenta D, et al. Transvenous implantable cardioverter-defibrillator (ICD) lead performance: a meta-analysis of Observational studies. J Am Heart Assoc 2015;4(11).

13. Link M, Sullivan RM, Olshansky B, et al. Implantable cardioverter defibrillator lead survival in athletic patients. Circ Arrhythmia Electrophysiol 2021;14(3).

14. NCAA banned Substances. Available at: https://www.ncaa.org/sports/2015/6/10/ncaa-banned-substances.aspx#:~:text=The%20NCAA%20bans %20the%20following,(banned%20for%20rifle% 20only. Accessed March 3, 2022.

15. Saarel E, Law I, Berul CI, et al. Safety of sports for young patients with implantable cardioverter-defibrillators: long-term results of the multinational ICD sports registry. Circ Arrhythmia Electrophysiol 2018;11(11):e006305.

16. Heidbuchel H, Willems R, Jordaens L, et al. Intensive recreational athletes in the prospective

17. James C, Bhonsale A, Tichnell C, et al. Exercise increases age-related Penetrance and arrhythmic risk in arrhthmogenic right ventricular dysplasia/cardiomyopathy associated desmosomal mutation carriers. J Am Coll Cardiol 2013;62(14).

18. Ruwald A-C, Marcus F, Estes III, et al. Association of competitive and recreational sport participation with cardiac events in patients with arrhythmogenic right ventricular cardiomyopathy: results from the North American multidisciplinary study of arrhythmogenic right ventricular cardiomyopathy. Eur Heart J 2015;36(27):1735–43.

19. Ommen S, Mital S, Burke MA, et al. AHA/ACC clinical practice guideline: 2020 AHA/ACC guideline for the diagnosis and treatment of patients with hypertrophic cardiomyopathy. Circulation 2020;142:e588–631.

20. Konhilas J, Watson PA, Maass A, et al. Exercise can prevent and reverse the severity of hypertrophic cardiomyopathy. Circ Res 2006;98(4):540–8.

21. Johnson JN, Ackerman Michael J. Return to play? Athletes with congenital long QT syndrome. Br J Sports Med 2013;47:28–33.

22. Ostby S, Bos JM, Owen HJ, et al. Competitive sports participation in patients with catecholaminergic polymorphic ventricular tachycardia: a single center's early experience. JACC Clin Electrophysiol 2016;2(3):253–62.

23. Kurtzwald-Josefson E, Hochhauser EK, Guy PE, et al. Exercise training improves cardiac function and attenuates arrhythmia in CPVT mice. J Appl Physiol 2012;113:1677–83.

24. Manotheepan R, Saberniak J, Danielsen TK, et al. Effects of Individualized exercise training in patients with catecholaminergic polymorphic ventricular tachycardia type 1. Am J Cardiol 2014;113(11):1829–33.

25. Kim J, Malhotra R, Chiampas G, et al. Cardiac arrest during long-distance running races. N Engl J Med 2012;366:130–40.

26. Baggish A, Battle RW, Beckerman JG, et al. Sports cardiology: core curriculum for providing cardiovascular care to competitive athletes and highly active people. J Am Coll Cardiol 2017;70:1902–18.

27. Wilkoff B, Hess M, Young J, et al. Differences in tachyarrhythmia detection and implantable cardioverter defibrillator therapy by primary or secondary prevention indication in cardiac Resynchronization therapy patients. J Cardiovasc Electrophysiol 2004;15(9):1002–9.

28. Investigators TAvIDA. A comparison of antiarrhythmic-drug therapy with implantable defibrillators in patients Resuscitated from Near-fatal

multinational ICD Sports Safety Registry: results from the European cohort. Eur J Prev Cardiol 2019;26(7):764–75.

ventricular arrhythmias. N Engl J Med 1997;337(22): 1576–1583A.

29. Investigators TC. Canadian implantable defibrillator study (CIDS)A Randomized trial of the implantable cardioverter defibrillator against amiodarone. Circulation 2000;101(11):1297–302.

30. Ruwald M, Ruwald A-C, Johanse JB, et al. Temporal incidence of appropriate and inappropriate therapy and mortality in secondary prevention ICD patients by cardiac diagnosis. JACC Clin Electrophysiol 2021;7(6):781–92.

31. Maron B, Zipes DP, Kovacs RJ. Eligibility and disqualification recommendations for competitive athletes with cardiovascular abnormalities: Preamble, Principles, and general considerations: a scientific statement from the American Heart Association and American College of Cardiology. Circulation 2015;132:e256–61.

32. Ackerman M, Zipes DP, Kovacs RJ, et al. Eligibility and disqualification recommendations for competitive athletes with cardiovascular abnormalities: task force 10: the cardiac channelopathies. Circulation 2015;132(22):e326–9.

33. Heidbuchel H, Arbelo E, D'Ascenzi F, et al. Recommendations for participation in lesiure-time physical activity and competitive sports of patients with arrhythmias and potentially arrhythmogenic conditions. Part 2: ventricular arrhythmias, channelopathies and implantable defibrillators. Eur Soc Cardiol 2021;23: 147–8.

34. Pelliccia A, Sharma S, Gati S, et al. 2020 ESC Guidelines on sports cardiology and exercise in patients with cardiovascular disease. Eur Soc Cardiol 2021; 42:17–96.

35. Lampert R, Zipes DP. Updated recommendations for athletes with heart disease. Annu Rev Med 2018;69:177–89.

36. Naik A, Kallen MA, Walder A, et al. Improving hypertension control in diabetes mellitus: the effects of collaborative and proactive health communication. Circulation 2008;117(11):1361–8.

37. Wilson SR, Strub P, Buist AS, et al. And the better outcomes of asthma treatment (BOAT) study group. Shared treatment decision making improves adherence and outcomes in poorly controlled asthma. Am J Respir Crit Care Med 2010;181:566–77.

38. Stacey D, Légaré F, Col NF, et al. Decision aids for people facing health treatment or screening decisions. Cochrane Database Syst Rev 2017;(4):CD001431.

39. Shapero K, Gier, Chad, et al. Experiences of athletes with arrhythmogenic cardiac conditions in returning to play. Heart Rhythm; 2022.

40. Nash D, Lee H-R, Janson C, et al. Video game ventricular tachycardia: the "Fortnite" phenomenon. Heart Rhythm Case Rep 2020;6(6):313–7.

41. Alkharaza A, Al-Harbi M, El-sokkari I, et al. The effect of revascularization on mortality and risk of ventricular arrhythmia in patients with ischemic cardiomyopathy. BMC Cardiovasc Disord 2020;20(455).

42. De Ferrari G, Dusi V, Spazzolini C, et al. Clinical management of catecholaminergic polymorphic ventricular tachycardia: the role of left cardiac sympathetic denervation. Circulation 2015;131(25): 2185–93.

43. Moss A, Schuger C, Beck CA, et al. Reduction in inappropriate therapy and mortality through ICD programming. N Engl J Med 2012;367(24):2275–83.

44. Kutyifa V, Daubert JP, Schuger C, et al. Novel ICD programming and inappropriate ICD therapy in CRT-D versus ICD patients: a MADID-RIT sub-study. Circ Arrhythmia Electrophysiol 2016;9(1).

45. Olshansky B, Atteya G, Cannom D, et al. Competitive athletes with implantable cardioverter–defibrillators—how to program? Data from the implantable cardioverter–defibrillator sports registry. Heart Rhythm 2019;16(4):581–7.

46. Slotwiner D, Varma N, Akar JG, et al. HRS Expert Consensus Statement on remote interrogation and monitoring for cardiovascular implantable electronic devices. Heart Rhythm 2015;12(7): e69–100.

47. Knops R, Nordkamp O, Delnoy PPHM, et al. Subcutaneous or transvenous defibrillator therapy. N Engl J Med 2020;383(6):526–36.

48. Schneider A, Burkhart HM, Ackerman MJ, et al. Minimally invasive epicardial implantable cardioverter-defibrillator placement for infants and children: an effective alternative to the transvenous approach. Heart Rhythm 2016;13(9):1905–12.

49. Parsons J, Anderson SA, Casa DJ, et al. Preventing catastrophic injury and death in collegiate athletes: Interassociation recommendations endorsed by 13 medical and sports medicine Organisations. J Athletic Train 2019;54(8):843–51.

The Tactical Athlete
Definitions, Cardiovascular Assessment, and Management, and "Fit for Duty" Standards

Jennifer Xu, MD[a], Mark C. Haigney, MD[b], Benjamin D. Levine, MD[c], Elizabeth H. Dineen, DO[a],*

KEYWORDS

- Tactical athlete • Military • Firefighter • Law enforcement • Cardiovascular screening

KEY POINTS

- Military, law enforcement, firefighters, and emergency response providers, referred to as tactical athletes, have a high demand for physical fitness and must endure mentally and physically demanding occupational tasks, often in extreme conditions.
- There is an increased risk for cardiovascular events when on duty rather than off duty.
- The tactical athlete is exposed to unique forms of cardiovascular stress and should be approached differently than a competitive athlete by the treating physician.
- In stress testing, efforts should be taken to simulate conditions encountered by the tactical athlete when assessing for "fit for duty" standards after a cardiac event.
- Medical decision-making regarding testing, treatment, and return to duty should be made in concert with the tactical athlete and a multidisciplinary team including key representatives understanding their discipline's governing policies.

INTRODUCTION

Understanding the physiologic demands and cardiac remodeling of competitive athletes has been a focus of clinical and research efforts to enable better cardiovascular care of this specialized population. Although some principles can translate to other athletic cohorts, it is important to differentiate the tactical athlete from the typical competitive athlete. Tactical athletes include the military, law enforcement, firefighters, and others whose physical training and responsibilities are centered not around competition but around service.

Although the absolute number of cardiovascular events is low in this population, there is an increased risk of cardiovascular events occurring on versus off the job, raising concerns about the cardiac risks of this line of work.

This article aims to (1) define tactical athletes and understand the cardiovascular demands of their specific jobs, (2) discuss what is known about cardiovascular disease management in this population, (3) outline cardiovascular testing protocols, and (4) highlight gaps in knowledge and suggest next steps to improve cardiovascular care for this population.

Disclosure Statement: The authors have nothing to disclose.
[a] University of California Irvine Medical Center, 333 City Boulevard West, Suite 400, Orange, CA 92868-3298, USA; [b] Military Cardiovascular Outcomes Research, Uniformed Services University, 4301 Jones Bridge Road, Bethesda, MD 20814, USA; [c] Institute for Exercise and Environmental Medicine, The University of Texas Southwestern Medical Center, 7232 Greenville Avenue, Suite 435, Dallas, TX 75231, USA
* Corresponding author.
E-mail address: dineene@hs.uci.edu

Cardiol Clin 41 (2023) 93–105
https://doi.org/10.1016/j.ccl.2022.08.008
0733-8651/23/© 2022 Elsevier Inc. All rights reserved.

DEFINITIONS

Tactical athletes are those who "use their minds and bodies to serve and protect individuals, communities, states, countries, and themselves,"[1] including military personnel, firefighters, law enforcement, emergency medical personnel, and others combating emergencies, accidents, natural disasters, and terrorist attacks. Tactical athletes must be ready to face any threat, whether physical, environmental, or psychological, often with little to no advanced notice. Their mission is distinct: "surviving and ensuring the survival of others."[2]

Distinction of a Tactical Athlete from a Competitive Athlete

To delineate how the tactical athlete population differs from the traditional athlete, the definition of a competitive athlete should be considered. According to the Bethesda guidelines, the competitive athlete is defined as "one who participates in an organized team or individual sport that requires competition against others as a central component, places a high premium on excellence and achievement, and requires some form of systematic (and usually intense) training."[3]

A tactical athlete also emphasizes occupational excellence and consistent training but the central component is service, rather than competition.[2] Call to duty for a tactical athlete can occur at any time; in contrast to traditional athletic competitions, with their designated schedules, tactical athletes are deployed to missions that can last for several days, often in environments with extremes of noise, temperature, humidity, and altitude. Many of the duties of a tactical athlete are physically unfavorable, potentially involving heavy lifting or maneuvering into difficult positions while wearing heavy gear. While on missions, tactical athletes have limited opportunities for recovery, at times enduring inadequate sleep superimposed on potentially suboptimal nutrition (**Box 1**).

To endure these challenges, tactical athletes must be adaptable and resilient. Conditions can change quickly for these individuals—a crowd can grow restless or a humanitarian operation can turn into a combat engagement—requiring tactical athletes to adapt to their dynamic, sometimes life-threatening environments. Failure to perform, because of health issues or otherwise, may jeopardize their own lives, the lives of their teammates and those who they serve and protect.

TRAINING DEMANDS OF THE TACTICAL ATHLETE

Tactical athletes need to attain baseline fitness standards depending on the chosen discipline.

Once selected, they undergo occupation-specific training programs, comprising weeks to months of strenuous physical and mental conditioning.[1,2,4]

Military

The 6 branches of the United States military comprise the Army, Marine Corps, Navy, Air Force, Coast Guard, and Space Force. There are also Special Forces teams, elite members of the military who have passed even more rigorous training and implement covert, challenging operations by air, land, or sea.[1] The military generally tests physical fitness semiannually with weekly or daily participation requirements in physical training.

In the military, the ability to maintain tactical proficiency while enduring mental and physical stresses is an important determinant of success. Soldiers are required to be agile, with the ability to change modalities at short notice. The United States Army uses a 3-phase training system consisting of initial conditioning, toughening, and sustaining phases following principles of precision, progression, and integration.[5] During basic training, recruits must be prepared for calisthenics, sprint and distance running, combat training, marching, obstacle course navigation, engagement skills, marksmanship, and load-carriage tasks.[2]

Marines are required to pass the Combat Fitness Test, a 300-yard course including sprinting, high and low crawling, dragging and carrying another Marine, grenade throwing, and ammunition resupply, all while performing these tasks in full combat utility uniforms. Thereafter, Marines must pass the Physical Fitness Test once a year, a test that consists of a 3-mile run, pull-ups or push-ups, and crunches. They are assessed on a

---

Box 1
Unique characteristics of the tactical athlete compared with the competitive athlete

1. Focus is on service rather than competition.

2. High demand for speed, strength, and agility in addition to endurance (burst type activity), though often intermittent.

3. Performance under life-threatening conditions, while carrying heavy gear and equipment.

4. May perform under environmental extremes (heat, cold, altitude, weather).

5. Some overlap with standard occupational medicine.

6. Outcome affects survival of athlete and others, not just score.

points system and must receive a high enough score to pass; a maximum score for a man would be 23 pull-ups, 115 crunches, and a 3-mile run in 18 minutes (10 miles/h). This running speed translates to a peak oxygen uptake (VO2max) of approximately 56 to 60 mL/min/kg for the average 70 to 75 kg individual, a level of fitness similar to a collegiate running back in American football or a soccer midfielder.[6] Marines are simply one example demonstrating how physical fitness requirements (**Table 1**) of each branch must adhere to different standards depending on the occupational need.[1]

Law Enforcement

Law enforcement comprises police, sheriff's patrol officers, detectives, criminal investigators, and correctional officers. Law enforcement constitutes a special occupational group with frequent workplace exposure to violence.[7] They are trained to execute their tasks quickly and deescalate provocative situations.[7] Licensing and training protocols for police officers in the United States vary by state and locale. The physical agility test before entry into police academy typically involves tasks such as obstacle course maneuvering, agility runs, body drag, and fence climbs.[8]

Firefighting

Firefighters extinguish hazardous fires and perform civilian rescue operations. They must wear heavy protective gear while carrying a variety of fire suppression equipment in high temperatures. Before entering an academy to pursue further training, firefighters are required to pass a physical ability test.[2] The test consists of 8 events including a stair climb, hose drag, equipment carry, ladder raise and extension, forcible entry, search, rescue, and ceiling breach and pull.[9] The events must be completed in less than 10 minutes 20 seconds in order for candidates to qualify for the academy.[9]

CARDIOVASCULAR ADAPTATIONS

The physiologic demands and expected cardiovascular adaptations of many types of tactical athlete are delineated in **Fig. 1**. Common exposures and related cardiovascular demands are listed here.

Episodic Exposure to Stimuli

A typical tactical athlete will encounter episodic surges of maximal work intensity without structured rest and recovery.[1] A member of the military may suddenly come on an ambush or a police officer may have to chase down a perpetrator on foot; such surges last for unpredictable amounts of time and recovery will not occur until the mission is deemed successful. These surges can lead to physical and mental exhaustion, speaking to the importance of pacing oneself. Although a tactical athlete cannot control most environmental factors, their training can aim to maximize their aerobic and anaerobic capacity as well as the metabolic economy of their tasks. This training will help them to understand their strengths and limitations so as to better physically and mentally pace themselves in the field.

The repeated exposure to stressors will result in increased catecholamine production, wherein heart rate, contractility, cardiac output, and pulmonary ventilation will increase in normal physiologic states in order to increase oxygen delivery to the muscles.[1] Even the threat of a stressor will produce marked changes in the cardiovascular system; sounding an alarm was found to increase firefighters' heart rates by an average of 47 beats per minute.[10] Similarly, on-duty police officers were found to have pronounced tachycardia during confrontational situations.[11]

These surges of intense physical exertion have been implicated in an increased risk of cardiovascular events. The relative risk of acute myocardial infarction is 2 to 10 times higher during vigorous physical exertion compared with other activities.[12] Submaximal to maximal physical exertion may trigger malignant cardiac arrhythmias and sudden cardiac death (SCD) in those at highest risk.[12] Importantly, the relative risk of SCD depends on the fitness of the individual, such that individuals engaging in habitual vigorous exercise have a lower risk of SCD during vigorous exertion. Although these data are startling, the sudden death event rate is quite low overall (1 sudden death per 1.51 million episodes of vigorous exertion).[13]

High-Altitude Environments

High altitudes are associated with reductions in the partial pressure of oxygen in the atmosphere, which will consequently lower the alveolar oxygen content and produce a state of relative hypoxia. The total amount of maximal oxygen uptake is expected to drop approximately 1% for every 100 m increase in altitude above 1500 m (ie, 10% decrease at 2500 m above sea level).[14] This relative decrease in maximal oxygen uptake is similar across age groups; however, if someone has a lower baseline functional capacity at sea level, then this drop may be accentuated at altitude.

Table 1
Physical fitness requirements and medical contraindications for tactical athletes

Tactical Athlete	Physical Ability Test Name	Examples of Tasks Required	Cardiac Conditions that Might Preclude Them from Participation	Governing Organization
US Marine Corps	Combat Fitness Test	800 yard movement to contact course, ammunition can lift, 300 yard shuttle run, maneuver under fire course	Any history of coronary artery disease, cardiomyopathy, recurrent syncope, a medical condition requiring an automatic implantable cardiac defibrillator due to ischemic or valvular disease, third-degree atrioventricular block, or heart transplant. Holding a prescription for an anticoagulant or antiplatelet agent, with the exception of aspirin, is also a disqualifying condition	US Marine Corps
US Army	Army Physical Fitness Test	Push-ups, sit-ups, 2-mile run	As above	US Army
US Navy	Physical Fitness Assessment	5-mile run, curl-ups, push-ups	As above	US Navy
US Air Force	Air Force Fitness Assessment	1.5-mile run, push-ups, sit-ups, cross-legged reverse crunches, or planks	As above, as well as pauses greater than 2.2 s, 3 or more beats of supraventricular tachycardia at a rate greater than 100, 3 or more beats of ventricular tachycardia, frequent ventricular premature beats, Wolff-Parkinson-White pattern demonstrating a PR interval less than 120 ms, left-axis deviation greater than	US Air Force

(continued on next page)

Table 1
(*continued*)

Tactical Athlete	Physical Ability Test Name	Examples of Tasks Required	Cardiac Conditions that Might Preclude Them from Participation	Governing Organization
			minus 45°, complete left bundle branch block, greater than moderate pulmonary, tricuspid, or mitral regurgitation, greater than mild aortic insufficiency, bicuspid aortic valve, mitral valve prolapse, or stenosis of any valve. Patients who hold a diagnosis of coronary artery disease and are only partially revascularized may lose their flight license. Medications of concern include anticoagulants, beta blockers (due to their negative side effects on G tolerance), and alpha blockers (due to risk of postural hypotension	
Special Forces	Upper Body Round Robin (for Tier 1 and Tier 2 Special Operations) Note: describes only one example of a test, as Special Forces are very diverse	1 min of pushups, 1 min of sit-ups, pull-ups, dips, bench press 80% bodyweight, 20-ft rope climb in body armor or weight vest, 1 min kip-ups, 4 × 25 m shuttle run, 5-mile run or 5-mile ruck march with 45-lb dry weight	As above	US Army
Law enforcement	Physical Efficiency Battery	Obstacle course with the following: climb a 7-ft slanted wall,	Pacemakers, prosthetic valves, any condition that requires the	US Federal Law Enforcement Training Center

(*continued on next page*)

Table 1 (continued)				
Tactical Athlete	Physical Ability Test Name	Examples of Tasks Required	Cardiac Conditions that Might Preclude Them from Participation	Governing Organization
		climb a horizontal rope 20 ft, traverse a horizontal rope 20 ft, jump a ditch measuring 6-ft wide and 12-in deep, run or walk across a 30-ft beam without falling off, jump or climb 2 4-ft walls, cross a horizontal ladder suspected 8 ft above the ground, crawl through a simulated covert, a climb a 20-ft vertical ladder	use of anticoagulant medication, coronary artery disease, hypertension that requires the use of any medication, left bundle branch block, myocarditis, endocarditis, pericarditis, valvular heart disease, dysrhythmias such as ventricular tachycardia or fibrillation, Wolff-Parkinson-White syndrome paroxysmal atrial tachycardia with or without block, cerebrovascular accident, pulmonary embolism within the past 6 months, cardiomyopathy from any cause, congestive heart failure, Marfan syndrome, congenital anomalies	
Firefighter	Candidate Physical Ability Test	Stair climb, hose drag, equipment carry, ladder raise and extension, forcible entry, search and rescue, ceiling breach and pull	Coronary artery disease, cardiomyopathy or congestive heart failure, acute pericarditis, endocarditis, or myocarditis, recurrent syncope, a medical requiring an automatic implantable cardiac defibrillator, history of	National Fire Protection Association

(continued on next page)

Tactical Athlete	Physical Ability Test Name	Examples of Tasks Required	Cardiac Conditions that Might Preclude Them from Participation	Governing Organization
Table 1 *(continued)*				
			ventricular tachycardia or ventricular fibrillation due to ischemic or valvular heart disease, or cardiomyopathy, third-degree atrioventricular block, cardiac pacemaker, hypertrophic cardiomyopathy, heart transplant	
Astronauts	Functional Fitness Assessment	Sit and reach, Smith bench press, leg press, pull-ups, push-ups, sliding crunches, stand test, hand grip test, cone agility test	Pericarditis, myocarditis, or endocarditis; major congenital abnormalities; evidence of CAD, MI, or angina; persistent tachycardia; arrhythmia; conduction defect; ECG abnormalities; thrombophlebitis; deep venous incompetence; varicose veins; peripheral vascular disease; cardiac tumor; valvular disorder or clinically significant hypertrophy; and dilation or reduced ejection fraction	National Aeronautics and Space Administration

Under hypoxic conditions, there will be a compensatory increase in sympathetic tone and concomitant vagal withdrawal. As a result, heart rate, stroke volume, and cardiac output will increase, at least acutely, increasing myocardial oxygen demand.[14] Hypoxia will also induce peripheral vasodilation, dropping the blood pressure acutely but eventually increasing in most individuals after acclimatization. Stroke volume also decreases early in the acclimatization process.

Hypoxia alone, or when combined with other environmental stressors such as temperature, exercise, dehydration, or injury, may precipitate an acute coronary syndrome. Additionally, mountainous locations are often in remote environments offering limited access to health care, which increases the likelihood of mortality from such cardiac events.[14] The risk of SCD for hiking (1 in 780,000) and downhill skiing (1 in 630,000) at altitude is 4-fold and 2-fold higher, respectively,

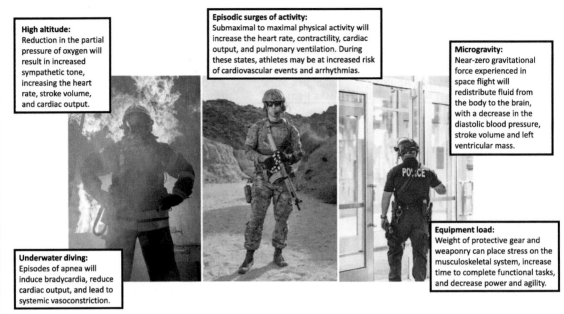

High altitude:
Reduction in the partial pressure of oxygen will result in increased sympathetic tone, increasing the heart rate, stroke volume, and cardiac output.

Episodic surges of activity:
Submaximal to maximal physical activity will increase the heart rate, contractility, cardiac output, and pulmonary ventilation. During these states, athletes may be at increased risk of cardiovascular events and arrhythmias.

Microgravity:
Near-zero gravitational force experienced in space flight will redistribute fluid from the body to the brain, with a decrease in the diastolic blood pressure, stroke volume and left ventricular mass.

Underwater diving:
Episodes of apnea will induce bradycardia, reduce cardiac output, and lead to systemic vasoconstriction.

Equipment load:
Weight of protective gear and weaponry can place stress on the musculoskeletal system, increase time to complete functional tasks, and decrease power and agility.

Fig. 1. Examples of potential tactical athlete occupational environmental conditions and their impact on the cardiovascular system.

than the sudden cardiac risk among the general population.[15] Acclimatization is suggested before exercise at altitude as a preventive measure.

Equipment Load

Most tactical athletes are required to carry heavy and unbalanced equipment, including protective gear, weaponry, and tools. A patrol officer is typically required to wear body armor weighing up to 8 lbs and carry approximately 20 lbs of equipment on their duty belt, including a weapon, ammunition, baton, flashlight, and handcuffs. Firefighter protective clothing and breathing apparatuses typically weigh more than 55 lbs, in addition to lifting and carrying loads in excess of 80 lbs.[16] Carrying heavy loads can contribute to physical injury, increase time to complete functional tasks, decrease power and agility, and increase perceived exertion.[16]

Underwater Diving

Tactical athletes will commonly carry a self-contained underwater breathing apparatus, or SCUBA, comprising a metal cylinder containing compressed air connected to a pressure regulator, to facilitate breathing underwater.[17] The most significant environmental exposure in diving is the increased ambient pressure that increases linearly the more the athlete descends. Breathing compressed air underwater results in increased dissolved inert gas in tissues and organs, such that on ascent, the dissolved gas can form gas bubbles in blood and tissues, and decompression sickness

can ensue if ascent is too rapid.[18] Furthermore, immersion in cold water can increase myocardial oxygen demand, increase central venous return, and induce peripheral vasoconstriction.[18]

Athletes may practice breath-hold diving, and these episodes of apnea will induce bradycardia, reducing cardiac output and increasing systemic vasoconstriction.[19] Careful attention must be paid to athletes with preexisting cardiac conditions, such as hypertension, coronary artery disease (CAD), bradyarrhythmia and tachyarrhythmia, that might be exacerbated by these periods of apnea.[19] The Centers for Disease Control cite a rate of occupational fatalities of 180 per 100,000 commercial divers per year, 40 times the mean rate for United States workers.[20] Death rates for military divers are unknown but due to the demands of service in this hostile environment, the selection criteria and training regimes for these elite forces are notoriously challenging.

Space

Tactical athletes who conduct missions in space, that is, astronauts, are exposed to decreased gravitational force, or microgravity. In microgravity, fluid is redistributed from the lower to the upper body, the carotid baroreceptors are reset, and a decrease in the diastolic blood pressure, stroke volume, and left ventricular mass are observed.[21] Although once thought that orthostatic hypotension might be a lasting effect of prolonged spaceflight, recent evidence has demonstrated that appropriate countermeasures, such as exercise training and appropriate volume resuscitation on return to Earth, can prevent clinically meaningful orthostatic intolerance.[22] Increased incidence of hypertension, CAD, or cardiac arrhythmias have not been convincingly implicated in athletes exposed to microgravity.[21]

Current Evidence on Cardiac Remodeling

Research on the specific type of cardiac remodeling encountered by tactical athletes is nascent and thus far data is limited. A Portuguese study subjected 76 candidates (men aged 20 to 24 years) for military special operations to a special training program composed of 20 hours of high intensity exercises. The exercises were a combination of primarily dynamic (long-distance running, long runs interspersed with sprinting and marching), primarily static (cargo transportation and weightlifting) and mixed exercises (steeplechase) and were designed to achieve periods of near maximal intensity (>96% of maximal heart rate). At the end of 25 weeks, they observed increases in left ventricular end-diastolic diameter (49.7 ± 3.2 to 52.8 ± 3.4 mm; $P < .01$) and left ventricular mass (93.1 ± 7.7 to 100.2 ± 11.4 g/m^2; $P < .01$), pretraining to posttraining, respectively.[23] The CHIEF study examined 1388 military men, aged 18 to 34 years, from the ROC Army Huadong Defense Command Base in Taiwan, and identified elite athletes as those who were able to perform military exercises one standard deviation above the mean. These individuals were found to have greater left ventricular mass index (84.4 ± 13.6 vs 80.5 ± 12.9 g/m^2, $P < .001$) and greater lateral mitral E'A' ratio (2.37 ± 0.73 vs 2.22 ± 0.76, $P < .01$) than those identified who were not elite.[24]

These studies revealed a significant increase in LV dimensions and mass consistent with eccentric remodeling in response to rigorous training programs. In the Portuguese study, 11.8% of subjects had eccentric hypertrophy after training compared to 5.9% pretraining.[23] Limitations to the studies were lack of controls and no long-term follow-up; furthermore, it is difficult to say whether the cardiac remodeling in training programs appropriately reflects longer term cardiac remodeling. As more disciplines are studied, the expected cardiovascular adaptations of each tactical athlete will be clarified more thoroughly.

CARDIOVASCULAR DISEASE IN THE TACTICAL ATHLETE–CURRENT EVIDENCE
Military

SCD is the most common nontraumatic cause of death in military recruits, and 86% occur during exertion.[25] The incidence of SCD in military recruits is estimated to be 13:100,000 recruit-years,[25] a number that is comparatively higher than the incidence of SCD in NCAA athletes (1:53,703 athlete-years),[26] raising concern that certain cardiac conditions are not adequately screened in this population. Regarding those on active duty, the 2020 study "Health of the Force for the US Army" found a prevalence of CAD of 5.7% to 6.7% and hypertension in 5.2% to 6.3% of the force between 2015 and 2019, compared to 21.6% and 21.2%, respectively, in the general population.[27,28]

Law Enforcement

A 2014 study found that up to 10% of all "on-duty" deaths for law enforcement officers were due to SCD.[29] Although physical restraints and altercations comprised about 1% to 2% of a police officer's annual professional time, they accounted for 25% of on-duty SCD.[29] This represents an SCD risk about 30 to 70 times higher than nonemergency law enforcement duties, although it should be emphasized that the absolute risk of cardiac events remains low. Similarly, although pursuits of suspects comprised less than 2% of on duty time, they were associated with 12% of SCD and risks 30 to 50 times higher than during nonemergency duties.[29] Hypertension is prevalent in the law enforcement population, ranging from 16% to 27%.[7] Dyslipidemia has been implicated in many active law enforcement officers with a prevalence significantly greater than that of the civilian population.[7]

Firefighting

A 2018 report by the National Fire Protection Association noted that 45% of on-duty firefighter fatalities were due to cardiovascular causes with the vast majority due to SCD[30] with an incidence rate of 18.1 deaths per 100,000 person-years.[31] A 2007 study examining causes of deaths of United States Firefighters between 1994 and 2004 found a 2.8-fold to 14.1-fold increase in sudden cardiac events during the alarm response period alone. The same study found that though fire suppression represents only about 1% to 5% of firefighters' professional time each year, 32% of deaths from CAD happened during this time, 10 to 100 times more common during emergency versus nonemergency duties. Cardiac events were more likely to occur in firefighters with risk factors for cardiovascular disease. Approximately 50% of firefighters have prehypertension, and 20% to 30% are hypertensive.[32]

In regards to arrhythmias in this population, a recent survey-based study of 10,860 firefighters demonstrated increased prevalence of atrial fibrillation that increased with numbers of fires fought per year; possible causation has been attributed to exposure to certain chemicals during firefighting.[33]

POSSIBLE EXPLANATION FOR INCREASED CARDIOVASCULAR RISK

These data suggest that the occupational duties of tactical athletes increase their risk of cardiovascular disease, possibly triggered by intense surges of physical activity and periods of high emotional stress. As the tactical athlete ages and becomes more sedentary, their risk factor profile starts to resemble that of the general population. Occupational exposure to excessive noise, smoke, as well as suboptimal working conditions such a poor diet and lack of sleep have also been cited as risk factors in the aging tactical athlete.[30] In a study of postmortem heart examinations, more frequent plaque ruptures were observed in those who died from an acute myocardial infarction during exertion when compared with those at rest.[22]

EVALUATION OF THE SYMPTOMATIC TACTICAL ATHLETE

Similar to diagnostic testing used to screen competitive athletes, cardiac testing for the symptomatic tactical athlete population prioritizes identifying high-risk conditions and ensuring pathologic diagnoses are differentiated from physiologic changes. If the incorrect evaluation takes place, then the life of the tactical athlete, the lives of his or her teammates, as well as the civilians they aim to protect, are at jeopardy. As such, the burden of proof for "fitness of duty" for the tactical athlete is often higher than for the competitive athlete.

The framework for the evaluation of a symptomatic tactical athlete is similar to a symptomatic competitive athlete and should begin with a careful history and physical examination to guide initial cardiac testing. It is essential to understand the individual tactical athlete's occupational requirements, providing context for testing and interpretation.

Many tactical athletes undergo regular screening stress testing. The testing should simulate the conditions of the tactical athlete as best as possible, ideally while wearing their tactical gear. Customized exercise protocols other than the standard Bruce protocol are recommended because the lifts, rucks, crawls, and other activities required of the tactical population are difficult to simulate with conventional exercise testing. For example, a customized stress test for a Marine, who must frequently handle heavy materials while crossing high obstacles, might involve performing sprints of maximal intensity while clothed in full gear, alternating with short rest periods.[34]

There is evidence to suggest that customized exercise testing can improve the diagnostic yield of exercise assessment following inconclusive graded exercise testing. Churchill and Wasfy identified 122 out of 1110 symptomatic patients who completed a graded exercise test but had unrevealing results, followed by additional customized exercise testing such as sprint intervals and race simulations.[35] Forty-eight of 122 (39%) patients had a "positive" (revealed actionable diagnosis or reproduced symptoms without clear diagnosis or pathology) customized test, unmasking a clinically actionable diagnosis in 26 of those 48 (54%). Effort should be made to diagnose or exclude potentially high-risk conditions as a cause for the tactical athlete's symptoms in order to facilitate safe return to work.

POLICIES GOVERNING "FITNESS FOR DUTY" AND RETURN TO DUTY AFTER A CARDIOVASCULAR EVENT

Every branch of the military publishes guidelines for medical fitness for duty, retention, and return to duty after a cardiac event. High-risk activities, such as aviation or special operations, have additional guidelines. Firefighters are bound by the National Fire Protection Association guidelines, and law enforcement officers have local guidelines available that can vary by city and state. Although there is variety among the different organizations, most trend toward relatively conservative guidelines surrounding fitness for duty. Some occupation-specific guidelines delineate specific requirements needed to achieve "medical clearance," for example, the National Fire Protection Association has suggested 12 METs as the minimum exercise capacity required for safe firefighting.

In brief, possession of certain preexisting cardiac conditions often equates to a disqualification (**Table 1**). These include history of CAD, cardiomyopathy, recurrent syncope, a medical condition requiring an automatic implantable cardiac defibrillator due to ischemic or valvular disease, third-degree atrioventricular block, or heart transplant.[36] Taking an anticoagulant or antiplatelet agent, with the exception of aspirin, is also commonly a disqualifying condition.[36]

For those who engage in flying duties, requirements are more stringent because a pilot's sudden incapacitation from a cardiovascular event could lead to a fatal crash. Disqualifying conditions include the above but also include many tachyarrhythmias and bradyarrhythmias and certain valvular heart diseases.[36] Medications of concern include anticoagulants, and antihypertensives that could have negative side effects on G-force tolerance or postural hypotension.[37]

Following the identification of a disqualifying condition, the medical provider will submit a summary to the qualifying medical board to see whether the individual meets requirements for a waiver. Medical waivers can be granted in some instances if the medical provider is able to prove that the condition does not pose a risk of sudden incapacitation or jeopardize occupational tasks, is nonprogressive, has low hemodynamic impact, and is able to be treated with medications that do not have any significant side effects precluding the individual from carrying out occupational tasks. Full disqualification is rare; in 2000, only 55 of almost 365,000 enlisted applicants (0.15%) to military service were found to be unfit because of cardiac or vascular disqualifications.

Once deemed low cardiovascular risk to return to duty, many tactical athletes will have a graded return under the guidance of their medical team. In the military, this "trial of duty" returns the military member to full service but does restrict them from performing vigorous physical exercises for a specific period. Their trial of duty begins when a cardiologist makes the recommendation that the individual is asymptomatic without objective evidence of ischemia with functional assessments such as stress testing. More specific recommendations are in place dependent on the medical condition/procedure. For pilots, when necessary, further return to duty evaluation can be pursued, including occupation-specific simulation testing such as centrifuge, altitude chambers, and motion simulation.[37,38]

Most of the medical decisions regarding a tactical athlete's return to duty after a cardiac event are at the discretion of the physician employed by the governing body with little input from the individual athlete impacted, and as such, medical decision-making is comparably more paternalistic than for the competitive athlete returning to play. Although the 2015 ACC/AHA/HRS eligibility and disqualification document for competitive athletes does place absolute disqualification for certain cardiac conditions such as hypertrophic cardiomyopathy (advice that continues to evolve over time), for conditions with more ambiguity it encourages a patient-centered approach in return to play decision-making by emphasizing counseling the individual athlete as well as engaging family members, the sponsoring school, and the athletic organization in the care of the athlete.[39] Furthermore, a more overt shared decision-making approach has been recommended in subsequent documents.[40]

Because of the potential for tactical athletes to experience unpredictable life-threatening situations at almost any time, most agree that it is better for tactical athletes to undergo a more conservative rehabilitative course before being released from treatment. In civilian occupations, such as law enforcement, this may take the form of a formal work-hardening program, a highly structured program individualized for each patient to gradually improve physical function and emulate on-the-job tasks. In military occupations, this will often involve a longer reconditioning phase with a focus on specific functional or tactical tasks associated with the service member's potential duties. It is imperative to engage all stakeholders throughout the medical decision-making process for any given tactical athlete so that the best decisions are made based on athlete's wishes and existing governing policies.

PREVENTION OF CARDIOVASCULAR DISEASE

Many fitness and wellness programs have now been adopted by each of the governing bodies in order to reduce the incidence of cardiovascular disease in tactical athletes. Blood pressure and lipids are regularly checked according to medical guidelines, and the triad of healthy diet, regular and frequent exercise, and good sleep hygiene is emphasized.

Coronary artery calcium score testing has emerged as a powerful noninvasive assessment in screening for CAD. In a healthy cohort of roughly 2000 active-duty army personnel, the presence of any amount of detectable coronary artery calcium increased cardiovascular events by nearly 12-fold.[38] The United States Air Force has been utilizing assessment of coronary artery calcium in its aviators since 1982.[41] In-house data derived from a cohort of almost 1500 aviators revealed that the presence of coronary artery calcium is most predictive of future cardiac events.[38] NASA has required coronary artery calcium scoring in its astronauts for more than a decade; the AstroCHARM calculator serves to help with risk prediction for cardiovascular disease.[42] Other organizations thus far have been slower to adopt coronary artery calcium scoring as regular practice.

DISCUSSION

An acute cardiovascular event in a tactical athlete poses a significant threat to the individual, the team, and overall success of the mission. However, there are several gaps in current knowledge in how to screen for and treat such events. Outcomes data on cardiovascular disease are not consistently collected in this population, especially in the military. There is very little research on arrhythmias in the tactical athlete population, which is a significant contributor to SCD. Very little is known about the specific cardiovascular remodeling that the tactical athlete population undergoes.

SUMMARY

Tactical athletes are individuals in the military, law enforcement, firefighting, and other professions whose occupations have significant physical fitness requirements coupled with the potential for exposure to frequent life-threatening situations while carrying heavy loads. Such exposures can have varied hemodynamic effects on the cardiovascular system. There is some evidence that engaging in tactical lines of work may increase the risk for sudden cardiac events, although future studies need to be conducted on this topic.

It is crucial that a clinical evaluation of the tactical athlete is inclusive of the individual's occupational requirements. Stress testing should consider the athlete's particular line of work and simulate their specific job duties as best as possible. Safety protocols regarding medical clearance for beginning and returning to work are relatively more stringent for this population than for competitive athletes due to the increased impact to the tactical athlete, their team, and the population they aim to serve and protect should they experience a cardiovascular event on the job. The task of the clinician asked to provide "clearance" for an individual to return to duty is complicated by the lack of consensus scientific statements similar to those of the Bethesda Conferences. Further research is needed to provide medical professionals with a standardized approach to these patients.

CLINICS CARE POINTS

- Military, law enforcement, firefighters, and emergency response providers, referred to as tactical athletes, have a high demand for physical fitness and must endure mentally and physically demanding occupational tasks, often in extreme conditions.

- There is an increased risk for cardiovascular events when on duty rather than off duty for tactical athletes.

- The tactical athlete is exposed to unique forms of cardiovascular stress and should be approached differently than a competitive athlete by the treating physician.

- In stress testing, efforts should be taken to simulate conditions encountered by the tactical athlete while on the job when assessing for return to work after a cardiac event.

- Medical decision-making regarding testing, treatment, and return to duty should be made in concert with the tactical athlete and a multidisciplinary team, including key representatives understanding their discipline's governing policies.

REFERENCES

1. Alver BA, Sell K, Deuster PA. NSCA's essentials of tactical strength and conditioning. 1st edition. Champaign (IL): Human Kinetics; 2017.
2. Scofield DE, Kardouni JR. The tactical athlete: a product of 21st century strength and conditioning. Strength Cond J 2015;37(4):2–7.
3. Mitchell JH, Maron BJ, Epstein SE. 16th Bethesda Conference: cardiovascular abnormalities in the athlete: recommendations regarding eligibility for competition. J Am Coll Cardiol 1985;6:1186–232.
4. Wise SR, Trigg SD. Optimizing health, wellness, and performance of the tactical athlete. Curr Sports Med Rep 2020;19(2):70–5.
5. Friedl KE, Knapik JJ, Kkinen KH, et al. Perspectives on aerobic and strength influences on military physical readiness: report of an international military physiology roundtable. J Strength Cond Res. 29(11S):S10-S23.
6. Astrand PO, Rodahl K, Dahl H, et al. Textbook of work physiology: physiological bases of exercises. 4th edition. Champaign (IL): Human Kinetics; 2003. p. 503–40.
7. Zimmerman FH. Cardiovascular disease and risk factors in law enforcement personnel: a comprehensive review. Cardiol Rev 2012;20(4):159–66.
8. Marins EF, Cabistany L, Farias C, et al. Effects of personal protective equipment on metabolism and performance during an occupational physical ability test for federal highway police officers. J Strength Cond Res 2020;34(4):1093–102.
9. Fyock-Martin MB, Erickson EK, Hautz AH, et al. What do firefighting ability tests tell us about firefighter physical fitness? A systematic review of the current evidence. J Strength Cond Res 2020;34(7):2093–103.
10. Smith DL, Manning TS, Petruzzello SJ. Effect of strenuous live-fire drills on cardiovascular and psychological responses of recruit firefighters. Ergonomics 2001;44:244–54.
11. Anderson GS, Litzenberger R, Plecas D. Physical evidence of police officer stress. Polic Int J Police Strateg Manag 2002;25(2):399–420.
12. Thompson PD, Franklin BA, Balady GJ, et al. Exercise and Acute cardiovascular events: placing the risks

into perspective: a scientific statement from the american heart association council on nutrition, physical activity, and metabolism and the council on clinical cardiology. Circulation 2007;115(17):2358–68.

13. Albert CM. Triggering of sudden death from cardiac causes by vigorous exertion. N Engl J Med 2000; 343(19):1355–61.

14. Cornwell WK, Baggish AL, Bhatta YKD, et al. Clinical implications for exercise at altitude among individuals with cardiovascular disease: a scientific statement from the american heart association. J Am Heart Assoc 2021;10(19):e023225.

15. Lo MY, Daniels JD, Levine BD, et al. Sleeping altitude and sudden cardiac death. Am Heart J 2013; 166(1):71–5.

16. Orr RM. Load carriage for the tactical operator: impacts and conditioning - a review. J Aust Strength Cond 2012;20(4):23–8.

17. Bove AA. Diving medicine. Am J Respir Crit Care Med 2014;189(12):1479–86.

18. Lynch JH, Bove AA. Diving medicine: a review of current evidence. J Am Board Fam Med 2009; 22(4):399–407.

19. Schagatay E, van Kampen M, Emanuelsson S, et al. Effects of physical and apnea training on apneic time and the diving response in humans. Eur J Appl Physiol 2000;82:161–9.

20. Centers for Disease Control and Prevention (CDC). Deaths associated with occupational diving–Alaska, 1990-1997. MMWR Morb Mortal Wkly Rep 1998; 47(22):452–5.

21. Vernice NA, Meydan C, Afshinnekoo E, et al. Long-term spaceflight and the cardiovascular system. Precis Clin Med 2020;3(4):284–91.

22. Fu Q, Shibata S, Hastings JL, et al. Impact of prolonged spaceflight on orthostatic tolerance during ambulation and blood pressure profiles in astronauts. Circulation 2019;140(9):729–38.

23. Dinis P, Dores H, Teixeira R, et al. Additional cardiac remodeling induced by intense military training in competitive athletes. Int J Cardiovasc Sci 2018; 31(3):209–17.

24. Liu PY, Tsai KZ, Lima JAC, et al. Athlete's heart in asian military males: the chief heart study. Front Cardiovasc Med 2021;8:1–829.

25. Eckart RE, Scoville SL, Campbell CL, et al. Sudden death in young adults: a 25-year review of autopsies in military recruits. Ann Intern Med 2004;141(11):829–34.

26. Harmon KG, Asif IM, Maleszewski JJ, et al. Incidence, cause, and comparative frequency of sudden cardiac death in national collegiate athletic association athletes: a decade in review. Circulation 2015;132(1):10–9.

27. 2020 health of the force (U.S. Army public health center website). 2020. Available at: https://phc.amedd.army.mil/PHC%20Resource%20Library/2020-hof-report.pdf. Accessed March 21, 2022.

28. Crawford AG, Cote C, Couto J, et al. Prevalence of obesity, Type II diabetes mellitus, hyperlipidemia, and hypertension in the United States: findings from the ge centricity electronic medical record database. Popul Health Manag 2010;13(3):151–61.

29. Varvarigou V, Farioli A, Korre M, et al. Law enforcement duties and sudden cardiac death among police officers in United States: case distribution study. BMJ 2014;349(nov18 2):g6534.

30. Kales SN, Soteriades ES, Christophi CA, et al. Emergency duties and deaths from heart disease among firefighters in the United States. N Engl J Med 2007; 356(12):1207–15.

31. Farioli A, Christophi CA, Quarta CC, et al. Incidence of sudden cardiac death in a young active population. J Am Heart Assoc 2015;4(6):e001818.

32. Smith DL, Barr DA, Kales SN. Extreme sacrifice: sudden cardiac death in the US Fire Service. Extreme Physiol Med 2013;2(6):1–9.

33. Vanchiere C, Thirumal R, Hendrani A, et al. Association Between Atrial Fibrillation and Occupational Exposure in Firefighters Based on Self-Reported Survey Data. 14. 2 (6), 1-9.

34. Sarma S, Levine BD. Beyond the bruce protocol: advanced exercise testing for the sports cardiologist. Cardiol Clin 2016;34(4):603–8.

35. Churchill TW, Disanto M, Singh TK, et al. Diagnostic yield of customized exercise provocation following routine testing. Am J Cardiol 2019;123(12):2044–50.

36. Department Of The Army Washington Dc. Medical services: standards of medical fitness. Defense Technical Information Center; 2002. https://doi.org/10.21236/ADA402408.

37. Nicol ED, Rienks R, Gray G, et al. An introduction to aviation cardiology. Heart 2019;105(Suppl 1):s3–8.

38. Davenport E, Palileo E, Gore S. Cardiovascular screening for pilots, aircrew, and high performance & spaceflight passengers. REACH 2021;21-22: 100040.

39. Levine BD, Baggish AL, Kovacs RJ, et al. Eligibility and disqualification recommendations for competitive athletes with cardiovascular abnormalities: task force 1: classification of sports: dynamic, static, and impact. Circulation 2015;132:e262–6.

40. Baggish AL, Ackerman MJ, Putukian M, et al. Shared decision making for athletes with cardiovascular disease: practical considerations. Curr Sports Med Rep 2019;18(3):76–81.

41. DeFina LF, Radford NB, Barlow CE, et al. Association of all-cause and cardiovascular mortality with high levels of physical activity and concurrent coronary artery calcification. JAMA Cardiol 2019;4(2):174–81.

42. Khera A, Budoff MJ, O'Donnell CJ, et al. Astronaut cardiovascular health and risk modification (Astro-CHARM) coronary calcium atherosclerotic cardiovascular disease risk calculator. Circulation 2018; 138(17):1819–27.

Exercise After Acute Myocarditis
When and How to Return to Sports

Robyn E. Bryde, MD[a], Leslie T. Cooper Jr, MD[a], DeLisa Fairweather, PhD[a,b],
Damian N. Di Florio, BS[a,b], Matthew W. Martinez, MD[c,*]

KEYWORDS

- Myocarditis • Return to play • Arrhythmia • Virus • Mitochondria • Sex differences • Exercise
- Cardiac magnetic resonance imaging

KEY POINTS

- Myocarditis is an inflammation of the myocardium with the most feared consequence being sudden cardiac death owing to arrhythmia.
- Cardiac MRI is an important diagnostic and prognostic tool for cases of symptomatic myocarditis.
- Guidelines recommend return to play following myocarditis no sooner than 3 to 6 months in addition to follow-up testing, which may include repeat cardiac MRI.

BACKGROUND

Sudden cardiac death (SCD) associated with sports participation is a tragic event, and much has been done to better understand and prevent this occurrence. Early studies evaluating SCD in athletes implicated hypertrophic cardiomyopathy as the most common cause of SCD in the United States.[1] However, more recent studies involving international data and the military have found normal autopsies in the majority of cases raising the possibility of yet undefined channelopathies and arrhythmia as a significant cause of SCD.[2–11] To date, approximately 6% to 14% of SCD events in athletes are attributed to myocarditis.[6,12] However, autopsy, which is needed to identify myocarditis, is not consistently performed, and the contribution of myocarditis to SCD may be underestimated. The mechanism by which myocarditis causes SCD in athletes is attributed to both focal cellular electrical instability and ischemia leading to polymorphic ventricular tachycardia or sometimes heart block.[13] National and international societies provide recommend timelines for return to play (RTP) after acute myocarditis to mitigate the risk of SCD.

DISCUSSION
Definition and Epidemiology

Myocarditis is an inflammation of the myocardium that occurs primarily in response to infectious agents but can also be caused by noninfectious insults, such as autoimmune disorders and/or inherited cardiomyopathies. Viral illnesses are most implicated with acute myocarditis worldwide except for *Trypanosoma cruzi* infection, leading to Chagas disease in South America. Adenovirus and enterovirus are the most likely infectious causes in the United States with parvovirus B-19 and human herpesvirus 6 currently most implicated in Europe.[14–16] More recently, SARS-CoV-2 and the messenger RNA (mRNA) vaccines used against the virus have been linked to the development of myocarditis.

The authors have nothing to disclose.

[a] Department of Cardiovascular Medicine, Mayo Clinic, 4500 San Pablo Road, Jacksonville, FL 32224, USA;
[b] Center for Clinical and Translational Science, Mayo Clinic, Rochester, MN 55902, USA; [c] Chanin T. Mast Hypertrophic Cardiomyopathy Center and Sports Cardiology, Atlantic Health, Morristown Medical Center, 111 Madison Avenue, Morristown, NJ, USA
* Corresponding author.
E-mail address: Matthew.Martinez@atlantichealth.org

Cardiol Clin 41 (2023) 107–115
https://doi.org/10.1016/j.ccl.2022.08.009
0733-8651/23/© 2022 Elsevier Inc. All rights reserved.

Myocarditis is defined as probable, possible, and definite based on the combination of symptoms and diagnostic test results. Possible myocarditis is defined with a high degree of certainty based on the following: (1) cardiac symptoms (dyspnea, chest pain, palpitations, syncope); (2) elevated cardiac troponin (cTn); (3) abnormal electrocardiogram (ECG) (diffuse T-wave inversions, ST-segment elevations without reciprocal ST-segment depressions, prolongation of the QRS duration), and/or abnormal echocardiogram (left ventricular wall motion abnormalities in a noncoronary distribution); and (4) abnormal cardiac magnetic resonance (CMR) imaging findings, such as late gadolinium enhancement (LGE) in a nonischemic pattern with prolonged native T1 and T2 relaxation times.[17] Possible myocarditis is defined when cardiac symptoms, elevated cTn, and abnormal ECG and/or echocardiographic findings are present with the absence of CMR or endomyocardial biopsy (EMB) evidence or the inability to perform CMR or EMB.[17] Definite myocarditis is defined by compatible histopathologic findings from endomyocardial or surgical biopsy or from autopsy specimens. When an acute pericarditis clinical syndrome and elevated troponin occur together, the condition is termed myopericarditis. Myocarditis specifically after vaccination may be defined according to the Brighton or Centers for Disease Control and Prevention criteria.[18,19]

Lake Louise criteria (LLC) help define CMR abnormalities for the diagnosis of myocarditis. LLC include CMR evidence of the following: (1) myocardial edema on T2-mapping sequences showing regional or global increases in native T2 and/or T2 signal intensity; (2) nonischemic myocardial injury with abnormal regional or global increases in native T1 or extracellular volume and/or regional LGE. Supportive findings on CMR that are not sufficient in themselves for diagnosis include the following: (1) pericardial effusion detected on cine CMR images; (2) pericardial inflammation with LGE, T1 or T2 mapping; and/or (3) LV wall motion abnormalities.[20]

Recently, several large cohort studies in athletes used the LLC to determine cardiac involvement by CMR to help define and identify cases of COVID-19 myocarditis. One study evaluating the risk of developing myocarditis after SARS-CoV-2 infection in young (≤20 years of age) otherwise healthy people found the incidence to be around 450 per million cases.[21] When CMR imaging was used as a screening tool to evaluate for cardiac involvement in acute and subacute COVID-19, approximately 2.3% of athletes had findings that met the updated 2018 LLC for clinical myocarditis.[22,23]

Although the LLC was originally developed for the diagnosis of myocarditis in symptomatic patients, these criteria were adapted to ascertain whether athletes had definite, probable, or possible myocarditis after COVID-19, despite many asymptomatic athletes. There was high variability among studies for the presence of cardiac involvement and of methods used to quantify and report myocardial tissue characterization. The studies used nonstandardized methods for CMR identification of cardiac involvement, and cardiac abnormalities did not meet LLC for myocarditis. Many of these studies did not include control groups of uninfected athletes for comparison. For post–vaccine myocarditis, the Centers for Disease Control and Prevention recently reported 1226 cases of probable myocarditis/pericarditis and 323 confirmed myocarditis/pericarditis cases after approximately 300 million COVID-19 mRNA vaccine doses, supporting a very rare occurrence of myocarditis/pericarditis associated with mRNA vaccine administration.[24]

Last, it is worthwhile to discuss autoimmune myocarditis and the potential for inherited cardiomyopathies to progress to fulminant myocarditis. Idiopathic giant cell myocarditis (GCM) is a rare and usually rapidly progressive form of autoimmune myocarditis generally found in younger men and women.[25] Although GCM may respond to immunosuppressive therapy with early diagnosis and treatment, the disease is often fatal secondary to life-threatening arrhythmias or cardiogenic shock.[25] A more chronic form of autoimmune myocarditis is idiopathic granulomatous myocarditis or sarcoid myocarditis. The incidence of cardiac involvement with pulmonary or systemic sarcoidosis is reported around 5%; however, this number is likely an underestimate of cases with histologic cardiac involvement.[26] Morbidity and mortality from sarcoid myocarditis are common and result from bradyarrhythmias or tachyarrhythmias and SCD.[27]

Inherited cardiomyopathies can lead to the development of myocarditis as evident in both premortem and postmortem studies.[28,29] Therefore, family screening may be beneficial for the early recognition and delivery of preventative therapies and/or treatments to this patient population, and exercise restrictions may be warranted owing to the genetic propensity for phenotypic expression with exposure to exercise. Arrhythmogenic right ventricular cardiomyopathy (ARVC) causes mutations in genes encoding desmosomal proteins and is most often acquired in an autosomal dominant pattern, which can lead to ventricular arrhythmias, ventricular dysfunction, and SCD.[30,31] In addition, initially introduced in 2008 by Sen-Chowdhry and colleagues,[32–34] there is growing evidence of arrhythmogenic left ventricular cardiomyopathy (ALVC) linked to gene mutations, which encode desmoplakin and Filamin C. The result is cardiomyocyte loss and repair with replacement by fibrofatty tissue, similar to what causes the arrhythmogenic milieu implicated in ARVC.[34,35] Fabry disease is an X-linked disease caused by deleterious mutations in the GLA (α-galactosidase A) gene and has a prevalence of about 1:117,000 in the general population.[36] Fabry myocarditis results from glycosphingolipid accumulation in cardiac myocytes, which generates a proinflammatory response from cardiomyocyte necrosis and fibrosis.[37]

Pathogenesis

The pathogenesis of viral myocarditis in mouse models and clinically can be divided into 3 phases: an early phase of viral entry into cells and activation of the innate immune response (develops in minutes to hours and is upregulated in the heart from day 3–5), activation of the adaptive immune response leading to acute myocarditis (which typically occurs in the first 7–14 days after infection), and a chronic phase that can last from months (in animal models and humans) to years (in humans), where remodeling and fibrosis progress to dilated cardiomyopathy (DCM) and chronic heart failure.[38–41] SARS-CoV-2 largely follows the same pattern, although the spike protein itself can persist in cells studied in vitro and cause myocyte dysfunction. The long-term clinical impact of these findings is under investigation.[42] GCM generally has an accelerated disease course with quick progression to heart failure and intractable ventricular arrhythmias. In comparison, inherited cardiomyopathies, such as Fabry disease and ARVC, are slowly progressive over time with symptoms developing after myocardial tissue is replaced by fibrosis or fibrofatty scar, respectively, similar to the progression to DCM after myocarditis.[15,38] The clinical presentation of arrhythmia varies greatly during myocarditis. During the acute phase of illness, arrhythmia is thought to be secondary to multiple factors, including the following: (1) direct cytotoxic effects leading to electrical instability from membrane dysfunction; (2) ischemia from macrovascular or microvascular and endothelial dysfunction; (3) gap junction dysfunction; and (4) abnormal calcium handling particularly with arrhythmogenic cardiomyopathies.[13] In contrast, arrhythmia presenting in the chronic DCM phase of disease is likely secondary to fibrosis and scar.[13]

There is currently no clear understanding of why viruses such as coxsackievirus (CVB), influenza, HIV, poliovirus, hepatitis C virus, or SARS-CoV-2 would target the heart or the mechanism for how these relatively mild viral cardiac infections lead to sex differences in heart failure. CVB3 has been shown to require mitochondria for viral replication,[43] and many of the viruses that cause myocarditis target mitochondria as part of their replicative cycle.[44–47] The abundant mitochondria required to meet the heart's high energetic demands provide an explanation for why such disparate types of viruses, that have no obvious cardiac tropism, would target the heart. Exercise typically improves cardiac function even after diseases such as ischemia[48,49]; however, during viral myocarditis, strenuous exercise increases the risk of SCD leading to the current guidelines recommending that patients abstain from exercise for 3 to 6 months after diagnosis.[12] Surprisingly, basic research animal studies conducted to understand the mechanisms that may account for SCD with myocarditis after exercise is around 30 years old.[50–53] These studies demonstrated increased mortality, viral titers, autoantibodies, and inflammation in animals with viral myocarditis after exercise.[50–53] More recently, exercise has been found to cause mitochondrial fission mediated by Drp1, while Drp1/fission is required for CVB3 replication.[54] In addition, b-adrenergic receptor activation also leads to mitochondrial fission of cardiac myocytes in culture,[54] providing a further possible mechanism for heart failure. Research is needed in this area, and the authors' laboratory (Fairweather) is examining the potential role of these pathways in increasing heart failure during viral myocarditis.[55]

Clinical Presentation

The clinical presentation of myocarditis is heterogeneous but generally includes cardiac symptoms, including chest pain, dyspnea, palpitations, heart failure, syncope, and rarely, SCD.[56] Exertional symptoms include exercise intolerance/fatigue, palpitations/tachycardia, or presyncope with return to exercise.[57] The disease can present at any age, but it is most frequently diagnosed in young adults.[56] When considering the diagnosis in the older adult population, it is imperative to rule out other causes of symptoms, such as coronary artery disease and/or anomalous coronary arteries with invasive coronary angiography or cardiac computed tomography angiography.

In general, myocarditis is considered acute when symptoms develop within 3 months and chronic when symptoms develop after 3 months of illness. There should be a high index of suspicion for viral myocarditis with the development of cardiac symptoms coinciding 1 to 4 weeks after viral illness. Following a new or recent diagnosis of SARS-CoV-2, development of cardiopulmonary symptoms at any time, particularly when returning to sports participation, should prompt further evaluation for myocardial involvement.[57] Although rare (0.5%–3.0%), cardiopulmonary symptoms of chest pain or dyspnea is considered an independent predictor of SARS-CoV-2 cardiac involvement in young healthy athletes.[22,23,58]

Diagnosis

Initial tests for clinically suspicious myocarditis should include the following: (1) a complete blood count, basic metabolic panel, cTn, C-reactive protein, and natriuretic peptide if heart failure is uncertain; (2) an ECG; and (3) an echocardiogram. If there is a clinical concern for arrhythmia, an ambulatory ECG monitor should be obtained. Elevated troponin, ECG abnormalities (diffuse T-wave inversions, ST-segment elevation without reciprocal ST-segment depression, prolongation of the QRS duration, arrhythmia, and/or heart block), and/or new echocardiographic abnormalities (ventricular dysfunction in a noncoronary distribution) should trigger additional studies, including CMR and/or EMB if clinically warranted. Application of the previously mentioned LLC when interpreting CMR may aid in the diagnosis of myocarditis. However, the gold standard for diagnosis is histopathologic evidence on EMB using Dallas or immunocytochemical criteria.[59] It should be noted that cardiac necrosis that is part of the Dallas criteria is not necessary for the development of myocarditis, fibrosis, or progression to DCM in translational animal models of myocarditis.[39,41] Although not routinely performed, EMB should be considered when all other causes of heart failure have been excluded, and there remains a likelihood that EMB will yield a diagnosis that will change prognosis or management.[60]

If sarcoid myocarditis is suspected, fluorodeoxyglucose-PET may be obtained for both the diagnosis and the monitoring response to therapy.[13] If GCM is suspected, EMB is the only test to provide a definitive diagnosis. For the inherited cardiomyopathies, the 2010 Task Force Criteria facilitate the diagnosis of ARVC by a point system for specific major and minor criteria, including the presence of structural abnormalities, histopathologic findings, repolarization abnormalities, depolarization abnormalities, arrhythmia, and family history.[31] However, these same criteria can lead to the misdiagnosis of left ventricular

arrhythmogenic cardiomyopathy. Therefore, genetic testing for mutations in the genes encoding desmoplakin, filamin C, and desmin may provide the most accurate means for the diagnosis of arrhythmogenic cardiomyopathies.[61] If Fabry disease is suspected, measurement of alpha-Gal A activity in men or gene analysis of the GLA gene may confirm diagnosis.[36]

Management

Most cases of myocarditis resolve in the first 2 to 4 weeks. However, approximately 25% of cases develop persistent symptoms, and 12% to 25% decompensate acutely and require advanced therapies.[56] Recent translational studies suggest benefits of a tailored therapy approach for specific causes of myocarditis in conjunction with guideline-directed medical care.[62] There should also be a low threshold for repeat testing with imaging or arrhythmia monitoring in patients with ongoing or worsening symptoms and/or for disease surveillance. Reliance on normalization of cardiac and inflammatory biomarkers to predict resolution of LGE on initial CMR should be correlated with caution, as 1 study reported an improvement in biomarkers and LGE on follow-up imaging, whereas a significant minority (21%) had worsening LGE despite normalization of cardiac biomarkers.[63] These data suggest that repeat CMR to assess the change in LGE may have unique prognostic value in the risk assessment of myocarditis.[63]

Mild to severe cases of myocarditis should initially be managed in a hospital setting, preferably one capable of providing advanced heart failure therapies. Treatment of heart failure is managed with standard therapies, including diuretics, ACE inhibitors, and beta-blockers. In patients with heart failure symptoms refractory to medical therapy or with hemodynamically significant arrhythmia, mechanical circulatory support may be used during the acute phase of illness or as a bridge to transplant. Arrhythmia is common and may respond to medications like class III antiarrhythmics. An implantable cardioverter-defibrillator (ICD) or pacemaker may be indicated in cases of sustained or symptomatic ventricular arrhythmia or high-grade conduction abnormalities, respectively. Temporary implanted devices are frequently used in the acute setting and transitioned to permanent devices if survival after the acute phase is expected to be greater than 1 year.[64]

The use of antiviral therapies for treatment of viral myocarditis is not yet established based on randomized clinical trial data.[25] Immunosuppressive agents may be considered in cases of fulminant myocarditis with biopsy evidence of severe inflammatory infiltrates.[65] However, the effect of such therapy in SARS-CoV-2 remains unknown. Firm evidence for the use of immunosuppressive therapies for the treatment of myocarditis is limited to use with GCM and sarcoid myocarditis. Treatment of GCM with immunosuppressive therapies includes steroids, cyclosporine, and sometimes azathioprine.[25] Treatment of sarcoid myocarditis is similar with first-line therapy-inducing steroids and second-line therapy with methotrexate.

Treatment of the inherited cardiomyopathies relies largely on supportive measures. Although less is known about the development of ALVC from desmoplakin mutations, emerging evidence suggests there is a greater propensity toward the development of myocarditis when compared with ARVC.[34] In general, therapies include medical management of heart failure symptoms, amiodarone, and beta-blocker use for arrhythmia, ICD for SCD prevention, and ultimately heart transplantation for the most refractory cases. In addition, restriction from sports participation is recommended for healthy gene carriers and individuals affected by the disease owing to the high risk of disease progression with exposure to exercise.[30,66] For Fabry disease, early diagnosis and consideration for enzyme replacement therapy (ERT) may prevent development of myocarditis. Although response to ERT after the development of Fabry myocarditis remains controversial, most experts agree ERT early in the disease course may prevent disease progression.[37,67]

Return to Play

The Task Force 3 criteria for return to sports following an acute clinical syndrome consistent with myocarditis recommend repeat evaluation no sooner than 3 to 6 months following the initial illness. At that time, athletes should undergo repeat testing with a resting echocardiogram, 24-hour Holter monitor, and exercise ECG. It is reasonable to RTP with normalization of systolic function, cardiac biomarker, and absence of arrhythmia on exercise ECG and/or Holter monitoring.[66] When doubt exists regarding resolution of inflammation based on cardiac testing or if symptoms persist or develop after RTP, there should be a low threshold for repeat CMR testing.[63,68] For patients with confirmed COVID-19 myocarditis, RTP following 3 months of exercise abstinence was deemed safe in a study with a 12-month follow-up period.[69]

It is important to address RTP strategies in the era of COVID-19 owing to the potential, albeit low likelihood of developing viral myocarditis.[22,23,58] Initial RTP strategies were more conservative and recommended a 10-day self-isolation with abstinence from exercise owing to concerns of clinical deterioration. However, follow-up studies demonstrating a lack of myocardial involvement in mild COVID-19 cases resulted in a recent update to the RTP guidelines by the American College of Cardiology Expert Consensus Decision Pathway.[17] New RTP recommendations include the following: (1) asymptomatic cases are recommended to abstain from exercise for 3 days to ensure symptoms do not develop; (2) mild or moderate cases with mild to moderate noncardiopulmonary symptoms are recommended to abstain from exercise until symptom resolution. No additional cardiac tests are required before RTP in these 2 clinical scenarios, but it is recommended that RTP begin with a graded regimen.

RTP recommendations differ for patients with cardiopulmonary symptoms and/or for patients diagnosed with severe COVID-19. These patients should undergo triad testing with ECG, cTn, echocardiogram, and cardiology consultation. If results of triad testing are normal, the athlete may RTP in a graded manner. If results to triad testing are abnormal or if symptoms develop after RTP, CMR and cardiology consultation is recommended. In patients with a prolonged COVID-19 course with symptoms beginning or lasting weeks to months after the initial infection, it is reasonable to perform triad testing and limit physical exercise. However, those with a prolonged course without cardiopulmonary symptoms are encouraged to resume a graded exercise regimen. In any of the above scenarios, if results to CMR testing reveal the presence of LGE, sports participation may be considered as part of shared decision making after cardiology consultation in the absence of systolic dysfunction, ventricular arrhythmia, and if cardiac biomarkers have normalized.[68]

Last, it should be noted that although CMR may be useful to guide diagnosis and prognosis, the routine use of CMR in the absence of concerning cardiopulmonary symptoms and/or abnormalities on prior cardiac tests is recommended against.[68] The application of CMR and the updated LLC to diagnose COVID-19 myocarditis in athletes with no symptoms of myocarditis and its use in RTP decision making require attention to detail. The use of CMR for myocarditis and outcome data involves symptomatic patients with inflammation largely limited to the heart. Most of the validation studies of myocarditis diagnosed on CMR have LGE, which has been validated more extensively than mapping abnormalities in histologically proven viral myocarditis. In populations with low prevalence of myocarditis, including healthy athletes, T1 and T2 mapping will have a low positive-predictive value. In addition, studies have shown adverse prognostic significance for LGE in patients with myocarditis,[70] and there are no prognostic data for abnormalities on T1 or T2 mapping in the absence of LGE. Finally, there are few data regarding T1 and/or T2 mapping abnormalities in the absence of LGE, including whether its present in exercising athletes, transformation into cardiac damage (fibrosis/scar), and any prognostic implications. There is a need to improve interpretation methods for CMR to quantify cardiac involvement in myocarditis, particularly as they pertain to T1 and T2 measures, which can be variable.

As for RTP strategies for the inherited cardiomyopathies, athletes with a definite, borderline, or possible diagnosis of ARVC should not participate in most competitive sports, and the prophylactic placement of an ICD to permit participation in high-intensity sports is not recommended.[66] However, it may be considered reasonable for these athletes to participate in low-intensity sports.[66]

SUMMARY

Myocarditis is an inflammatory disease of the myocardium secondary to infectious or noninfectious causes. Although the disease is generally mild, the most feared consequences include heart failure, arrhythmia, and SCD. Early recognition is essential for optimal short- and long-term outcomes, and accurate diagnosis often relies heavily on cardiac imaging with CMR and appropriate application of the LLC for interpreting imaging abnormalities. Most therapies for myocarditis are considered supportive and focus on the treatment of heart failure and arrhythmia with directed medical therapy. Treatment with immunosuppressive agents is often reserved for specific cases, including GCM and sarcoid myocarditis. Management strategies also include abstinence from exercise in the short term with specific RTP recommendations instituted after 3 to 6 months following a comprehensive cardiovascular evaluation, which includes triad testing (echocardiogram, 24-hour Holter monitor, and exercise ECG). CMR as part of an RTP strategy is warranted if abnormalities are present on follow-up testing or if symptoms develop after reinstating an athlete. However, the routine use of CMR as part of an RTP strategy in asymptomatic athletes is generally recommended against.

CLINICS CARE POINTS

- Myocarditis is an inflammatory disease of the myocardium of infectious or noninfectious etiology
- Although mild in most cases, it is a recognized etiology for heart failure, rhythm disturbance and sudden death.
- Most require only abstinence from exercise with return to play strategies based on cardiac imaging, stress testing and ambulatory monitoring.
- CMR plays an integral role in diagnosis, risk stratification and prognosis but is not part of routine RTP strategies in those who are asymptomatic.

DISCLOSURES/FUNDING

The authors have no financial or other disclosures. The work has been performed with support from National Institutes of Health (NIH) grant TL1 TR002380 (to D.N. Di Florio and D. Fairweather) and National Institute of Allergy and Infectious Diseases (NIAID) grants R21 AI145356, R21 AI152318, R21 AI154927, National Heart Lung and Blood Institute (NHLBI) grant R01 HL164520, and American Heart Association grant 20TPA35490415 (to D. Fairweather).

REFERENCES

1. Maron BJ, Doerer JJ, Haas TS, et al. Sudden deaths in young competitive athletes: analysis of 1866 deaths in the United States, 1980–2006. Circulation 2009;119(8):1085–92.
2. Corrado D, Basso C, Rizzoli G, et al. Does sports activity enhance the risk of sudden death in adolescents and young adults? J Am Coll Cardiol 2003; 42(11):1959–63.
3. Eckart R, Shry E, Burke A, et al. Department of Defense Cardiovascular Death Registry G. Sudden death in young adults: an autopsy-based series of a population undergoing active surveillance. J Am Coll Cardiol 2011;58(12):5.
4. Eckart RE, Scoville SL, Campbell CL, et al. Sudden death in young adults: a 25-year review of autopsies in military recruits. Ann Intern Med 2004;141(11): 829–34.
5. Harmon KG, Asif IM, Maleszewski JJ, et al. Incidence, cause, and comparative frequency of sudden cardiac death in national collegiate athletic association athletes: a decade in review. Circulation 2015;132(1):10–9.

6. Harmon KG, Asif IM, Maleszewski JJ, et al. Incidence and etiology of sudden cardiac arrest and death in high school athletes in the United States, . Mayo Clin Proc. 11th91. Elsevier; 2016. p. 1493–502. https://doi.org/10.1016/j.mayocp.2016.07.021.

7. Harmon KG, Drezner JA, Maleszewski JJ, et al. Pathogeneses of sudden cardiac death in national collegiate athletic association athletes. Circ Arrhythmia Electrophysiol 2014;7(2):198–204.

8. Holst AG, Winkel BG, Theilade J, et al. Incidence and etiology of sports-related sudden cardiac death in Denmark—implications for preparticipation screening. Heart Rhythm 2010;7(10):1365–71.

9. Papadakis M, Sharma S, Cox S, et al. The magnitude of sudden cardiac death in the young: a death certificate-based review in England and Wales. Europace 2009;11(10):1353–8.

10. Puranik R, Chow CK, Duflou JA, et al. Sudden death in the young. Heart rhythm 2005;2(12):1277–82.

11. Solberg EE, Gjertsen F, Haugstad E, et al. Sudden death in sports among young adults in Norway. Eur J Prev Cardiol 2010;17(3):337–41.

12. Maron BJ, Thompson PD, Ackerman MJ, et al. Recommendations and considerations related to preparticipation screening for cardiovascular abnormalities in competitive athletes: 2007 update: a scientific statement from the American Heart Association Council on Nutrition, Physical Activity, and Metabolism: endorsed by the American College of Cardiology Foundation. Circulation 2007;115(12):1643–55.

13. Peretto G, Sala S, Rizzo S, et al. Arrhythmias in myocarditis: state of the art. Heart Rhythm 2019; 16(5):793–801.

14. Mahrholdt H, Wagner A, Deluigi CC, et al. Presentation, patterns of myocardial damage, and clinical course of viral myocarditis. Circulation 2006; 114(15):1581–90.

15. Jain A, Norton N, Bruno KA, et al. Sex differences, genetic and environmental influences on dilated cardiomyopathy. J Clin Med 2021;10(11):2289.

16. Kuhl U, Pauschinger M, Noutsias M, et al. High prevalence of viral genomes and multiple viral infections in the myocardium of adults with "idiopathic" left ventricular dysfunction. Circulation 2005;111(7):887–93.

17. Committee W, Gluckman TJ, Bhave NM, et al. 2022 ACC expert Consensus decision pathway on cardiovascular sequelae of COVID-19 in adults: myocarditis and other myocardial involvement, post-acute sequelae of SARS-CoV-2 infection, and return to play: a report of the American College of cardiology solution set oversight committee. J Am Coll Cardiol 2022; 79(17):1717–56. https://doi.org/10.1016/j.jacc.2022.02.003.

18. Tejtel SKS, Munoz FM, Al-Ammouri I, et al. Myocarditis and pericarditis: case definition and guidelines for data collection, analysis, and presentation of immunization safety data. Vaccine 2022;40(10):1499–511.

19. Clinical considerations: myocarditis and pericarditis after receipt of mRNA COVID-19 vaccines among adolescents and young adults. Available at: https://www.cdc.gov/vaccines/covid-19/clinical-considerations/myocarditis.html. Accessed May 23, 2022.

20. Ferreira VM, Schulz-Menger J, Holmvang G, et al. Cardiovascular magnetic resonance in nonischemic myocardial inflammation: expert recommendations. J Am Coll Cardiol 2018;72(24):3158–76.

21. Singer ME, Taub IB, Kaelber DC. Risk of myocarditis from COVID-19 infection in people under age 20: a population-based analysis. medRxiv 2021.

22. Daniels CJ, Rajpal S, Greenshields JT, et al. Prevalence of clinical and subclinical myocarditis in competitive athletes with recent SARS-CoV-2 infection: results from the big ten COVID-19 cardiac registry. JAMA Cardiol 2021;6(9):1078–87.

23. Moulson N, Petek BJ, Drezner JA, et al. SARS-CoV-2 cardiac involvement in young competitive athletes. Circulation 2021;144(4):256–66.

24. Tom Shimabukuro M, MPH MBA. COVID-19 vaccine safety updates advisory committee on immunization practices (ACIP). 2021. Available at: https://www.cdc.gov/vaccines/acip/meetings/downloads/slides-2021-06/03-COVID-Shimabukuro-508.pdf. Accessed February 15, 2022.

25. Cooper LT Jr, Berry GJ, Shabetai R. Idiopathic giant-cell myocarditis—natural history and treatment. N Engl J Med 1997;336(26):1860–6.

26. Birnie DH, Nery PB, Ha AC, et al. Cardiac sarcoidosis. J Am Coll Cardiol 2016;68(4):411–21.

27. Ekström K, Lehtonen J, Nordenswan H-K, et al. Sudden death in cardiac sarcoidosis: an analysis of nationwide clinical and cause-of-death registries. Eur Heart J 2019;40(37):3121–8.

28. Groeneweg JA, Bhonsale A, James CA, et al. Clinical presentation, long-term follow-up, and outcomes of 1001 arrhythmogenic right ventricular dysplasia/cardiomyopathy patients and family members. Circ Cardiovasc Genet 2015;8(3):437–46.

29. Cooper LT Jr, Čiháková D. Do genes influence susceptibility to myocarditis? Washington DC: American College of Cardiology Foundation; 2021. p. 593–4.

30. Corrado D, Link MS, Calkins H. Arrhythmogenic right ventricular cardiomyopathy. N Engl J Med 2017;376(1):61–72.

31. Marcus FI, McKenna WJ, Sherrill D, et al. Diagnosis of arrhythmogenic right ventricular cardiomyopathy/dysplasia: proposed modification of the task force criteria. Circulation 2010;121(13):1533–41.

32. Sen-Chowdhry S, Syrris P, Prasad SK, et al. Left-dominant arrhythmogenic cardiomyopathy: an

under-recognized clinical entity. J Am Coll Cardiol 2008;52(25):2175–87.

33. Ortiz-Genga MF, Cuenca S, Dal Ferro M, et al. Truncating FLNC mutations are associated with high-risk dilated and arrhythmogenic cardiomyopathies. J Am Coll Cardiol 2016;68(22):2440–51.

34. Smith ED, Lakdawala NK, Papoutsidakis N, et al. Desmoplakin cardiomyopathy, a fibrotic and inflammatory form of cardiomyopathy distinct from typical dilated or arrhythmogenic right ventricular cardiomyopathy. Circulation 2020;141(23):1872–84.

35. Corrado D, Marra MP, Zorzi A, et al. Diagnosis of arrhythmogenic cardiomyopathy: the Padua criteria. Int J Cardiol 2020;319:106–14.

36. Zarate YA, Hopkin RJ. Fabry's disease. Lancet 2008; 372(9647):1427–35.

37. Frustaci A, Verardo R, Grande C, et al. Immune-Mediated myocarditis in Fabry disease cardiomyopathy. J Am Heart Assoc 2018;7(17):e009052.

38. Schultheiss H-P, Fairweather D, Caforio AL, et al. Dilated cardiomyopathy. Nat Rev Dis primers 2019; 5(1):1–19.

39. Coronado MJ, Brandt JE, Kim E, et al. Testosterone and interleukin-1β increase cardiac remodeling during coxsackievirus B3 myocarditis via serpin A 3n. Am J Physiology-Heart Circulatory Physiol 2012; 302(8):H1726–36.

40. Onyimba JA, Coronado MJ, Garton AE, et al. The innate immune response to coxsackievirus B3 predicts progression to cardiovascular disease and heart failure in male mice. Biol Sex Differences 2011;2(1):1–13.

41. Tschöpe C, Ammirati E, Bozkurt B, et al. Myocarditis and inflammatory cardiomyopathy: current evidence and future directions. Nat Rev Cardiol 2021;18(3): 169–93.

42. Navaratnarajah CK, Pease DR, Halfmann PJ, et al. Highly efficient SARS-CoV-2 infection of human cardiomyocytes: spike protein-mediated cell fusion and its inhibition. J Virol 2021;95(24):e01368-21.

43. Robinson SM, Tsueng G, Sin J, et al. Coxsackievirus B exits the host cell in shed microvesicles displaying autophagosomal markers. PLoS Pathog 2014;10(4): e1004045.

44. Gannagé M, Dormann D, Albrecht R, et al. Matrix protein 2 of influenza A virus blocks autophagosome fusion with lysosomes. Cell Host & Microbe 2009; 6(4):367–80.

45. Kim S-J, Syed GH, Khan M, et al. Hepatitis C virus triggers mitochondrial fission and attenuates apoptosis to promote viral persistence. Proc Natl Acad Sci 2014;111(17):6413–8.

46. Kyei GB, Dinkins C, Davis AS, et al. Autophagy pathway intersects with HIV-1 biosynthesis and regulates viral yields in macrophages. J Cell Biol 2009; 186(2):255–68.

47. Taylor MP, Kirkegaard K. Modification of cellular autophagy protein LC3 by poliovirus. J Virol 2007; 81(22):12543–53.

48. Fiuza-Luces C, Delmiro A, Soares-Miranda L, et al. Exercise training can induce cardiac autophagy at end-stage chronic conditions: insights from a graft-versus-host-disease mouse model. Brain Behav Immun 2014;39:56–60.

49. Fukuta H, Goto T, Wakami K, et al. Effects of exercise training on cardiac function, exercise capacity, and quality of life in heart failure with preserved ejection fraction: a meta-analysis of randomized controlled trials. Heart Fail Rev 2019;24(4):535–47.

50. Hosenpud JD, Campbell SM, Niles NR, et al. Exercise induced augmentation of cellular and humoral autoimmunity associated with increased cardiac dilatation in experimental autoimmune myocarditis. Cardiovasc Res 1987;21(3):217–22.

51. Kiel R, Smith F, Chason J, et al. Coxsackievirus B3 myocarditis in C3H/HeJ mice: description of an inbred model and the effect of exercise on virulence. Eur J Epidemiol 1989;5(3):348–50.

52. Reyes MP, Lerner AM. Interferon and neutralizing antibody in sera of exercised mice with coxsackievirus B-3 myocarditis. Proc Soc Exp Biol Med 1976; 151(2):333–8.

53. Tilles JG, Elson SH, Shako JA, et al. Effects of exercise on coxsackie A9 myocarditis in adult mice. Proc Soc Exp Biol Med 1964;117(3):777–82.

54. Coronado M, Fajardo G, Nguyen K, et al. Physiological mitochondrial fragmentation is a normal cardiac adaptation to increased energy demand. Circ Res 2018;122(2):282–95.

55. Di Florio DN, Sin J, Coronado MJ, et al. Sex differences in inflammation, redox biology, mitochondria and autoimmunity. Redox Biol 2020;31:101482.

56. Caforio AL, Pankuweit S, Arbustini E, et al. Current state of knowledge on aetiology, diagnosis, management, and therapy of myocarditis: a position statement of the European Society of Cardiology Working Group on Myocardial and Pericardial Diseases. Eur Heart J 2013;34(33):2636–48.

57. Petek BJ, Moulson N, Baggish AL, et al. Prevalence and clinical implications of persistent or exertional cardiopulmonary symptoms following SARS-CoV-2 infection in 3597 collegiate athletes: a study from the Outcomes Registry for Cardiac Conditions in Athletes (ORCCA). Br J Sports Med 2021;56(16): 913–8.

58. Martinez MW, Tucker AM, Bloom OJ, et al. Prevalence of inflammatory heart disease among professional athletes with prior COVID-19 infection who received systematic return-to-play cardiac screening. JAMA Cardiol 2021;6(7):745–52.

59. Cooper LT Jr. Myocarditis. N Engl J Med 2009; 360(15):1526–38.

60. Yancy CW, Jessup M, Bozkurt B, et al. 2013 ACCF/AHA guideline for the management of heart failure: executive summary: a report of the American College of Cardiology Foundation/American Heart Association Task Force on practice guidelines. Circulation 2013;128(16):1810–52.

61. Corrado D, Zorzi A, Cipriani A, et al. Evolving diagnostic criteria for arrhythmogenic cardiomyopathy. J Am Heart Assoc 2021;10(18):e021987.

62. Tschöpe C, Cooper LT, Torre-Amione G, et al. Management of myocarditis-related cardiomyopathy in adults. Circ Res 2019;124(11):1568–83.

63. Berg J, Kottwitz J, Baltensperger N, et al. Cardiac magnetic resonance imaging in myocarditis reveals persistent disease activity despite normalization of cardiac enzymes and inflammatory parameters at 3-month follow-up. Circ Heart Fail 2017;10(11):e004262.

64. Al-Khatib SM, Stevenson WG, Ackerman MJ, et al. 2017 AHA/ACC/HRS guideline for management of patients with ventricular arrhythmias and the prevention of sudden cardiac death: a report of the American College of cardiology/American heart association task force on clinical practice guidelines and the heart rhythm society. J Am Coll Cardiol 2018;72(14):e91–220.

65. Kociol RD, Cooper LT, Fang JC, et al. Recognition and initial management of fulminant myocarditis: a scientific statement from the American Heart Association. Circulation 2020;141(6):e69–92.

66. Maron BJ, Udelson JE, Bonow RO, et al. Eligibility and disqualification recommendations for competitive athletes with cardiovascular abnormalities: task force 3: hypertrophic cardiomyopathy, arrhythmogenic right ventricular cardiomyopathy and other cardiomyopathies, and myocarditis: a scientific statement from the American Heart Association and American College of Cardiology. J Am Coll Cardiol 2015;66(21):2362–71.

67. Weidemann F, Niemann M, Störk S, et al. Long-term outcome of enzyme-replacement therapy in advanced Fabry disease: evidence for disease progression towards serious complications. J Intern Med 2013;274(4):331–41.

68. McKinney J, Connelly KA, Dorian P, et al. COVID-19–myocarditis and return to play: reflections and recommendations from a Canadian working group. Can J Cardiol 2021;37(8):1165–74.

69. Patriki D, Baltensperger N, Berg J, et al. A prospective pilot study to identify a myocarditis cohort who may safely resume sports activities 3 months after diagnosis. J Cardiovasc Translational Res 2021;14(4):670–3.

70. Georgiopoulos G, Figliozzi S, Sanguineti F, et al. Prognostic impact of late gadolinium enhancement by cardiovascular magnetic resonance in myocarditis: a systematic review and meta-analysis. Circ Cardiovasc Imaging 2021;14(1):e011492.

Printed and bound by CPI Group (UK) Ltd, Croydon, CR0 4YY

03/10/2024

01040363-0007